Diagnosis:
HEART DISEASE

Answers to Your Questions
about Recovery and Lasting Health

Diagnosis:
HEART DISEASE

███

ANSWERS TO
YOUR QUESTIONS
ABOUT RECOVERY AND
LASTING HEALTH

John W. Farquhar, M.D.
Gene A. Spiller, Ph.D.

W. W. Norton & Company
New York   London

The table on page 21–22 is from *The American Way of Life Need Not Be Hazardous to Your Health*, revised edition, by J. W. Farquhar, copyright © 1987 by the Stanford Alumni Association. Reprinted by permission of Perseus Books Publishers, a member of Perseus Books, L.L.C.

For information about permission to reproduce selections from this book, write to Permissions, W. W. Norton & Company, Inc., 500 Fifth Avenue, New York, NY 10110

The text of this book is composed in Berkeley with the display set in Futura
Composition by AW Bennett Inc.
Manufacturing by the Haddon Craftsmen, Inc.

Library of Congress Cataloging-in-Publication Data

Farquhar, John W., 1927–
Diagnosis—heart disease : answers to your questions about recovery and lasting health / John W. Farquhar, Gene A. Spiller
p.   cm.
Includes bibliographical references and index.
ISBN 0-393-05012-2
1. Coronary heart disease—Popular works. 2. Coronary heart disease—Patients—Rehabilitation. 3. Coronary heart disease—Prevention. I. Spiller, Gene A. II. Title.

RC685.C6 F365 2001
616.1'23—dc21   00-062210

ISBN 0-393-32235-1 pbk.

W. W. Norton & Company, Inc., 500 Fifth Avenue, New York, N.Y. 10110
www.wwnorton.com

W. W. Norton & Company Ltd., Castle House, 75/76 Wells Street, London W1T 3QT

1 2 3 4 5 6 7 8 9 0

Contents

—

Acknowledgments

Many people—too many to be mentioned—have contributed to our present knowledge of heart disease, and it is their work that has made this book possible. Many of them had a vision that went beyond their time.

The first acknowledgment must go to Bonnie Bruce, Dr.P.H., R.D., of the Sphera Foundation, who made a major contribution to the book. Donna Louie, R.N., and Sallie Whaley, R.N., of the Cardiac Therapy Foundation of the Mid-Peninsula in Palo Alto, California, who have dedicated many years to cardiac rehabilitation, made important contributions to Chapter 7. Christine Reicker assisted us with her knowledge of fitness exercises, and John Richards, a Palo Alto artist, provided the artwork.

We are thankful to Rosemary Schmele of the Sphera Foundation for proofreading, for making valuable editing suggestions on the entire manuscript, and for help in word processing, and to Mora Dewey and Connie Burton for editorial assistance.

We also thank our many colleagues at the Stanford Center for Research in Disease Prevention for their numerous research contributions, many of which form the scientific underpinnings of this book.

And finally, we thank Nomi Victor of W. W. Norton for her editorial work on the manuscript, and Amy Cherry of W. W. Norton, who saw that we could write a different and creative book on this topic. Amy reminds us of some of the great book editors of the past. This book would not have been possible without her.

John W. Farquhar
Stanford, California

Gene A. Spiller
Los Altos, California

Introduction

For most people with heart disease the chances not only of survival but of a bright future that allows enjoyment of life at its fullest are greater today than ever before. Great strides have been made in both the treatment and prevention of heart disease. The death rate from coronary heart disease (CHD), which causes about half of all heart disease deaths, has decreased by about 55 percent since 1967. The rate of death from stroke has decreased even more. While improvements in medical technology are a large factor in these statistics, the good news for you, the patient, is that we now know that changes in diet, exercise, and smoking habits can alter, and even reverse, the course of a large number of cases of heart disease. Even for those with cardiovascular damage substantial enough that a return to a full and active life is unlikely, further damage can often be prevented.

Almost all diagnosed heart disease is really *artery* disease, where the arteries become clogged from blood cholesterol and prevent necessary oxygen, carried by the bloodstream, from reaching the heart. A whole host of secondary events can result: heart attack, congestive heart failure, stroke, and irregular heart rhythms. This arterial clogging—called *atherosclerosis*—today can be ameliorated by modern medical techniques *and also by changing our habits*.

You may have bought this book for one of these reasons:

- You have had a heart attack
- Your physician has given you a diagnosis of heart disease
- You have experienced symptoms which you suspect might indicate heart disease and want to go to your physician prepared to ask the right questions
- There is a history of heart disease in your family and you want to do all you can to prevent you and your relatives from developing it
- A friend or family member is confused about this disease and you feel this book may help
- You just want to know more about heart disease in order to prevent it

This book will answer all the above needs using as little jargon as possible.

The book is divided into two sections: one addressing immediate concerns if you have an ailment; the other showing how to implement a long-term, heart-healthy life plan. Part I of the book, "The Ailing Heart," describes the various heart diseases and symptoms, the workings of the heart, and the medical tests and treatments available to you, and helps you evaluate your risk factors for heart disease. Part II, "The Healthy Heart Lifestyle," helps you rethink the lifestyle options you have chosen.

The term "heart disease" is sometimes confusing, encompassing, as it does, a broad range of diseases that are sometimes not at all similar to one another, and symptoms that are not really diseases. We have organized this book so that you can quickly find what is relevant to your particular situation. If you want only a description of a symptom or disease and information about the tests and treatments available but do not want to know about the mechanics of the heart, skip Chapter 1. If you want to know about the mechanisms by which the heart functions and malfunctions, the information is available in Chapter 2. If you care primarily about risk and protective factors, read Chapter 3. Diagnostic tests are covered in Chapter 4, medications for heart disease in Chapter 5, major heart interventions from bypass to angioplasty in Chapter 6, and the crucial period for recovery after a heart attack in Chapter 7. If your main concern is prevention, read Part II of the book (Chapters 8–11 and the Epilogue). At the end of the book you'll find an extensive list of other books on the subject of heart disease, prevention, and lifestyle changes. This book will answer many commonly asked questions, and you'll also find questions to bring to your physician and other health care providers. You'll learn that many risk factors can be controlled by changing your lifestyle.

This brings us to the purpose of this book: of course, we wish to inform you, the patient, about the mechanisms and manifestations of heart disease, but *primarily we wish to educate you about the possibilities of actively participating in the prevention of and recovery from atherosclerotic heart disease.* It is with this intention that we have conceived the material in Part II, "The Healthy Heart Lifestyle."

You probably know that heart disease is the leading cause of death in the United States. In the United States and in industrialized countries like Canada, Britain, Germany, northern Italy (the industrial part of Italy), and central and eastern Europe, coronary heart disease (a narrowing of the coronary arteries surrounding the heart, usually due to atherosclerosis and frequently resulting in heart attack) is the most common type of heart disease. These countries have in common a certain degree of industrialization, sedentary living, cigarette smoking, and a diet rich in animal products and refined foods low in fiber. On the bright side, while heart disease is still the major killer in these Western countries, its *rate* is declining, especially in Britain, the United States, and Canada. On the dark side, rates are high and still increasing in eastern Europe; and as the Western way of life moves into Asia, Africa, and developing countries around the world, the heart disease rate climbs in these places as well. This is an indication that something in the Western way of life is to blame. In the United States a decrease in smoking, together with diet and exercise awareness, has been a major factor in the declining rate of heart disease deaths. Because of increasing health awareness and advances in medical intervention techniques, although the United States was once first, today it ranks tenth in heart disease deaths among major industrialized countries.

There are many cultural and psychological reasons why people fall into unhealthy habits, and habits are often difficult to change. However, a diagnosis of heart disease is serious, frightening, and potentially deadly. It can be a much needed wake-up call that shocks us into taking stock of our options and choosing those that will not only improve our health but lead us toward wholeness in our lives.

PART I

THE AILING HEART

1

How the Heart Works

The heart as a pump

The heart is a pump that rhythmically contracts and relaxes. Think of the principles at work in a hand-operated water pump. When the handle is depressed, pressure is put on the water and it exits through a spigot. When the handle is raised, a vacuum is created and water is drawn in from the well. The flow of the water forces open a little "trap door," a valve, which opens in one direction only. Once the water is drawn up into the pumping apparatus, it cannot flow backward into the well, only outward to the spigot.

This is the way the heart works. It is the pump in charge of circulating oxygen, water, and nutrients through the bloodstream to all of the body's tissues, including its own. The heart wall is a muscle, and just like any other muscle, it needs oxygen, water, and nutrients to function. But unlike other muscles—for example, the ones in the arms or legs, which, when resting, need only a little oxygen—the heart muscle needs a good supply of oxygen every second of your life, in order to continue beating. The heart beats about 70 times each minute, sometimes faster, if you are physically active. (This means that the heart of an eighty-five-year-old person has beaten

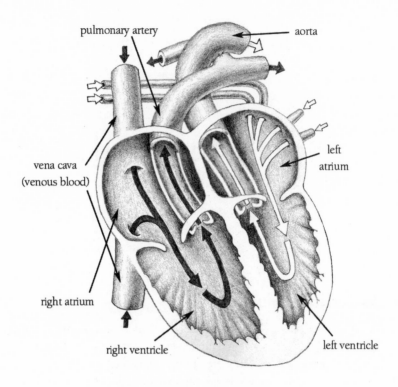

Figure 1-1. Cross section of the heart

over 3,127,320,000 times!) The more active you are, the greater your need for oxygen.

Two pumps in one

The heart is actually a *double* pump, each side quite distinct from the other. In this cross section of the heart (Figure 1-1) we see that there are four chambers. The two chambers on the right side receive blood returning from all parts of the body through a very large vein, the *vena cava*. This blood enters the top chamber, called the right *atrium* (*atrium* is a Latin word meaning the first room or chamber entered in a house); from here it goes to the lower chamber, the right *ventricle*, from which it is pumped through the pulmonary artery to the lungs to exchange its carbon dioxide for fresh oxygen.

This fresh blood, ready to feed oxygen to all the tissues, comes back to the left side of the heart, goes into the upper chamber, the left *atrium*, then down through a valve to the left *ventricle,* which pumps blood into the *aorta,* a very large artery that then subdivides into many smaller and smaller arteries throughout the body. The left side of the heart is completely separate from the right side.

The contraction phase of the heart is called *systole,* and the relaxation phase, when the chambers expand, drawing blood into the atria and ventricles, is called *diastole.*

The heart as part of the cardiovascular system

The heart is linked to the lungs by major blood vessels to allow for a continuous exchange of oxygen and for the elimination of carbon dioxide, the by-products of body energy production. Blood vessels, from large to very small, reach each tissue of the body. The vessels— you could call them pipes—that bring oxygen-rich blood from the lungs to the various parts of the body are called *arteries.* When the arteries become very small, they are called *capillaries,* a name derived from the Latin *capillus,* meaning hair, because the capillaries are as fine as human hair. The blood vessels that return blood from the tissues to the lungs are called *veins.*

The coronary arteries

Arteries forming a crown around the heart muscle bring oxygen and other nutrients to the heart. Because of their crownlike shape, they have been called *coronary arteries* (*corona* in Latin means crown). The coronary arteries are the lifeline that supplies what the heart needs to stay alive. Just as if you stop breathing for longer than a few moments, you suffocate and die, so the heart muscle cannot be without an open lifeline for more than a few minutes without suffering damage.

The heart valves

There are four valves in the heart, which prevent backward blood flow after the chambers contract and send blood forward to the ventricles, the pulmonary arteries, and the aorta. These valves are the *tricuspid valve,* which controls blood flow from the right atrium to the

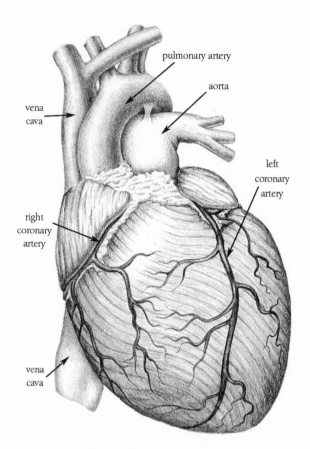

Figure 1-2. Coronary arteries

right ventricle; the *pulmonary valve*, which is the gate between the right ventricle and the pulmonary artery; the *mitral valve*, which allows blood to pass from the left atrium to the left ventricle; and the *aortic valve*, which allows blood to pass out from the left ventricle to the aorta.

The electrical system

All the pumping of the heart is controlled by a finely tuned electrical system. Let's return to the point where oxygen-depleted blood returns to the right side of the heart, into the *right atrium*. The right atrium also contains an electrical signal generator called the *sinoatrial node* (SA node). This node acts as a kind of natural pacemaker: it releases regular electrical impulses, which cause the right atrium to contract. (Remember, the heart is primarily a muscle, and its response to an electrical impulse is to contract.) Impulses from the brain, traveling through the nervous system, also affect the timing of the SA node's signal, but it has been found that the node can operate on its own if necessary.

When the electrical signal reaches the muscle of the atrium, the whole chamber contracts, forcing the blood inside the chamber past the tricuspid valve and into the right ventricle. The electrical impulse contacts another electrical node, the *atrioventricular node* (AV node), and stimulates the ventricle to contract, now forcing blood into the pulmonary arteries and toward the lungs. Almost simultaneously the left atrium and then the left ventricle contract, forcing oxygenated blood into the arteries to circulate through the body. This entire cycle of signal transmission and contraction of the heart's chambers (with ensuing relaxation as well) takes only about one second! You can see that if the electrical signal malfunctions, it can affect the entire blood and oxygen pumping system.

Blood pressure

Blood pressure is controlled mainly by the contraction and relaxation of the heart muscle, the shape and size of arteries, and proper kidney function. The most important cause of high blood pressure is constriction of the many miles of small arteries, called *arterioles*. The kidneys also affect blood pressure since they control the amount of fluids in the body by retaining or excreting water and certain minerals in solution in the blood, such as potassium and sodium; when water is retained, the volume of blood increases and this causes blood pressure to rise. Increased fluid volume *and* arteriole constriction are additive and raise blood pressure even more.

How the heart can break down

Damage to any one of the components of the heart can cause it to lose pumping efficiency, resulting in insufficient delivery of oxygen to various organs and especially to the heart itself. Breakdowns can occur in the delivery of electrical signals to the heart muscle; in the mechanical pumping action of the heart, including malfunctioning of the heart valves; and in the coronary arteries that make up the circulatory network of blood vessels that feed the heart muscle.

2

The Many Faces of Heart Disease

In this chapter you will find the answers to your questions about the major types of heart disease and their underlying causes like atherosclerosis. You will learn about the link between blood cholesterol and plaques in your arteries, coronary heart disease and heart attacks, arrhythmias, TIAs, heart block, and fibrillation. There will be a brief definition of a stroke, even though a stroke is not a disease of the heart, because the two share some similarities in their underlying causes. Of the diseases you will find in this chapter, what is called *coronary heart disease* is by far the most prevalent one.

What is heart disease?

The term "heart disease" refers to a group of heart and artery disorders that are part of a broader group called cardiovascular disease (cardio = heart, vascular = relating to blood vessels). These disorders are by far the largest cause of death in the United States in both men and women (about 1 million per year—*or one death every 33 seconds*). Over 90 percent of heart diseases are caused by one underlying problem—narrowing of the heart arteries by cholesterol and fibrous tissue, a process known as atherosclerosis.

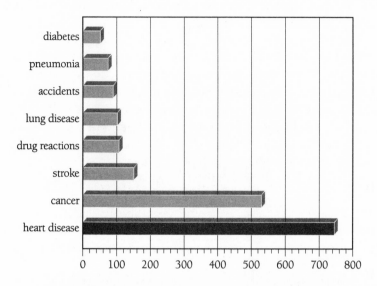

Figure 2-1. Major causes of death in the United States in 1994
(in thousands)

What is cholesterol?

Cholesterol is a waxy, fatlike substance produced by the liver, present in all animal tissue. It is an important substance with many functions in the body. It is a building block of cells, the starting molecule for the synthesis of many hormones—including sex hormones—as well as bile acids (produced by the liver and secreted into the intestines during a meal to help digest fats) and many other substances, like vitamin D.

When cholesterol is found in foods, it is referred to as *dietary cholesterol*. Dietary cholesterol is present in animal foods—meat, fish, eggs, and dairy products. When we eat food containing cholesterol, this cholesterol is absorbed from the intestines into the bloodstream. The cholesterol found in the blood is a combination of the cholesterol absorbed from food and the cholesterol synthesized by the liver. This is what is measured when you have a blood test and is referred to as *serum cholesterol* or *blood cholesterol*. Even though we call one dietary cholesterol and the other serum cholesterol, the cholesterol molecule is the same in both cases.

Plants do not have any cholesterol, but the cells of all plants contain similar substances called phytosterols (from *phytos*, the Greek word for plant). Phytosterols are not absorbed by the body and will actually block some of the cholesterol in your diet from being absorbed—which is one of the many reasons plant-based diets are healthful.

Your body makes all the cholesterol you need. If your diet contains too much additional cholesterol, your blood cholesterol levels will go up, contributing to your risk of atherosclerosis.

Is arteriosclerosis the same as atherosclerosis?

The words are almost interchangeable, but the word atherosclerosis is now used more commonly. *Arterio* means something that belongs to an artery, and *athero* means something gruel-like, soft, and pasty.

What does it mean that I have plaque in an artery in my heart?

Plaques are deposits of cholesterol and fibrous tissue built up over many years, beginning in childhood, in response to factors like smoking, high blood cholesterol, and high blood pressure, among others. These deposits are like lumps on the inside of the artery and are called atherosclerotic plaques. When the plaques build up and narrow the heart artery (known as a coronary artery) to about 50 percent of its original size, then the diagnosis of coronary artery disease may be made, although sensitive tests that are not often performed can detect smaller deposits.

After about 50 percent narrowing has occurred, coronary artery disease, also known as coronary heart disease, or CHD, can gradually or suddenly interfere with the pumping and circulation of blood, depriving tissue and organs (including the heart itself) of essential blood and oxygen.

I was told that I have coronary heart disease; what risks does this pose?

Frequently, if untreated, coronary heart disease leads to a "heart attack," also known as a myocardial infarction (an MI), or coronary

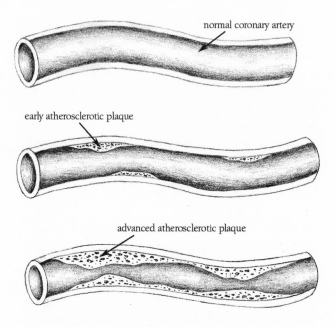

normal coronary artery

early atherosclerotic plaque

advanced atherosclerotic plaque

Figure 2-2. Various stages of atherosclerotic plaque forming in
coronary artery

thrombosis, which is fatal in about 30 percent of cases. About
1.5 million heart attacks occur each year. Hearts damaged by an MI,
especially if accompanied by high blood pressure (which is usually
called hypertension), can also result in weakened heart muscles and
a condition known as congestive heart failure, or CHF. Although
CHF causes about 50,000 deaths per year, CHD deaths are much
more frequent—about 500,000 per year.

The coronary heart disease and congestive heart failure varieties
of heart disease make up over 95 percent of all the heart disease in
the United States. The good news is that both diagnosis and treatment have improved dramatically over the past forty years, and a diagnosis of heart disease is no longer a reason to drop everything and
put your affairs in order. Rather, it is a call to mobilize your resources,
learn about your condition, and work with your doctors and health
professionals to arrest, treat, and, in some cases, reverse the disease.

Is angina "heart disease"?

Angina, called angina pectoris by doctors, is a symptom of under-lying coronary heart disease. It is caused by the narrowing of the heart arteries due to atherosclerosis, and is present in about 7 million Americans, with about 400,000 new cases yearly. Angina pectoris refers to the aching and gripping pain that occurs in the area under the breastbone in the central part of the chest, and it may extend to the jaw or to the left shoulder and arm. This pain, usually lasting less than five minutes, occurs most typically in response to exercise, and is more common on exposure to cold, after meals, or during stressful moments.

What does unstable angina mean?

Your doctor will term your angina "stable angina" if it comes at predictable times over a few weeks, but will refer to it as "unstable angina" if the pain comes at rest, is more severe, or increases in duration (over ten minutes) or frequency. Unstable angina is a signal that you need to seek immediate medical attention, as it may be the warning symptom of an impending heart attack.

What exactly is a heart attack?

A heart attack is a closure of one or more of the heart's arteries (the coronary arteries) sufficient to damage some heart muscle cells. The closure is due first to narrowing of the artery by atherosclerotic plaques, followed by a clot (or thrombus) that completely closes the artery, causing the usual "heart attack."

A heart attack, sometimes referred to as a "coronary," has two interchangeable "official" names: either *coronary thrombosis* or *myocardial infarction* (the latter often called MI). Since *thrombosis* means "clot," the term *coronary thrombosis* refers to the clot that blocks an artery. The narrowing of the artery makes it susceptible to a clot. The myocardial infarction is the end result: the heart muscle (the *myocardium*), now starved for oxygen because blood is no longer reaching some of the muscle, responds with an *infarction*. The term infarction is derived from a Latin word *infarcire* meaning "to stuff in"—referring to the reddish and swollen appearance of that injured part of the heart.

The closure of an artery by the thrombosis injures the heart's muscle cells, which release some chemicals, called enzymes, into the bloodstream, allowing your doctor to help confirm the diagnosis by measuring the levels of these enzymes.

What are the warning signs of a heart attack?

Heart attacks usually cause chest pain lasting more than ten minutes. They may also cause an abnormally rapid heartbeat, sweating, and, if severe, a loss of the heart's pumping action—leading to shock. Some milder heart attacks can occur without symptoms, and some may cause symptoms that are experienced as "indigestion" or a full feeling in the upper part of the abdomen.

What does my doctor mean if she says I have heart failure?

Heart failure, where the thickened heart muscle begins to lose its power to contract, is called congestive heart failure, or CHF. The word congestion is derived from the coughing and fluid buildup in the lungs that results from backward pressure caused by the weakened heart muscle. Congestive heart failure can be mild or severe, can cause shortness of breath, retention of water, ankle swelling—all evidence that the heart muscle has been weakened.

What is heart block?

Heart block is a partial or complete block of the electrical impulses originating in the atrium or sinus node preventing the electrical impulses from reaching the atrioventricular node and ventricles. There are various degrees of heart block. Heart block is often corrected by the use of a pacemaker (see Chapter 6).

If I have had a stroke, does this mean that I have heart disease?

No. A stroke means you have had damage to a part of the brain caused either by bleeding from a brain artery or from a blockage of a brain artery. Since it involves arteries, a stroke is an example of the vascular group of cardiovascular diseases. Strokes cause about 160,000

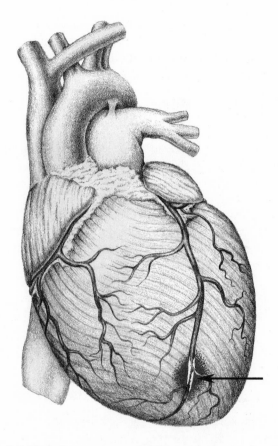

Figure 2-3. Blocked coronary artery in left ventricle showing damaged heart muscle, a myocardial infarction

deaths per year, or one every 3.3 minutes—about one fourth as many as are caused by coronary artery disease.

What causes strokes?

About two thirds of strokes are due to atherosclerotic plaques in the arteries of the brain (the *cerebral* arteries) which close down an artery by more than half and cause a blood clot to form that blocks the artery completely—this is what is known as a cerebral thrombosis. There are three main cerebral arteries: the *anterior*, *middle*, and *pos-*

terior cerebral arteries. Blockages due to clots occur in these major arteries or in their smaller branches. Strokes can also be caused by bleeding from a tear in the brain's arteries—these are called hemorrhagic strokes and are particularly common in those with high blood pressure.

My mother has a diagnosis of TIAs — what is that?

TIAs stands for transient ischemic attacks, often simply called "small strokes" in that their effects are often brief, usually lasting less than an hour. They may come repeatedly over a few days or weeks and are an important signal to seek medical care. Symptoms often include a brief numbness, tingling, or weakness on only one side of the body, or a temporary loss of the ability to speak. Most are caused by a small part of an atherosclerotic plaque breaking off from inside an artery that supplies blood to the brain and then moving "downstream." When one of these small fragments plugs an even smaller artery in the brain, it is called an embolis. The damage caused by a small fragment of a plaque lodging in a small artery in the brain is usually less severe for two reasons: the artery is small and doesn't supply a large section of the brain, and the material plugging the artery tends to dissolve within a few minutes.

My husband has an arrhythmia. Is that serious?

Arrhythmias are a disorder of the rhythm of the heartbeat, which can sometimes be life-threatening. Atrial fibrillation (in the upper chambers of the heart) is a type of arrhythmia that can be either converted to normal rhythm with an electrical shock to the heart or slowed by medicines. Atrial fibrillation results in an irregular pulse, usually at a pulse rate between 100 and 140. Any rapid, irregular heartbeat requires medical attention within a few hours. Atrial fibrillation becomes more common in people over fifty years of age. The real *cause* of atrial fibrillation is usually unknown, but some cases occur in people with overactive thyroid glands (known as thyrotoxicosis). Atrial fibrillation is not the *result* of coronary artery disease, but it can aggravate preexisting congestive heart failure, which itself is often caused by coronary artery disease.

An arrhythmia affecting the lower chambers of the heart (the ventricles) is very dangerous. The body can withstand ventricular fibrillation for only a few minutes before death occurs. Ventricular fibrillation is thought to be the immediate cause of most sudden deaths from heart disease. An arrhythmia, such as ventricular fibrillation, is almost always the *result* of a heart attack, usually occurring within minutes after the heart attack begins. The closure of a heart artery by a clot (the cause of a heart attack) deprives the heart muscle of blood and oxygen, triggering the ventricle to fibrillate—and losing its capacity as a pump as a result.

There are many different types of arrhythmias. Recent research has shown that diets containing omega-3 fats (such as flaxseed, walnuts, grape seeds, pumpkin seeds, sesame, salmon, tuna) will decrease the occurrence of sudden death due to arrhythmias. (See Chapter 11, page 124.) Some arrhythmias are the result of coronary artery disease, some result from transient "insults" to the heart from alcohol or drugs like cocaine. Certain arrhythmias in young people are due to inborn defects in the heart's complex electrical system. Any unusual type of heartbeat deserves medical attention so that a diagnosis can be made.

My grandmother had rheumatic heart disease. Is that the same as coronary heart disease?

No. It comes from the late effects of an earlier infection with the streptococcus bacteria called rheumatic fever, which was much more common fifty years ago, before antibiotics were available. Rheumatic fever damages one or more of the heart's valves. Modern cardiac surgery is now able to fix these valves and return a person to a nearly normal state of health.

My granddaughter was born with a congenital heart problem. Does this run in families?

No. About 30,000 babies are born each year with these heart defects. Since many of these can be fixed by surgery, only about 5,000 deaths per year result from these problems.

Can I inherit family traits that lead to heart disease?

The most common genetic abnormality that underlies *severe* heart disease (often called "premature heart disease"), which can occur even in ages as young as thirty years, is a condition where the total blood cholesterol is usually over 300 and the low-density cholesterol is over 220. (See Chapter 3 for a discussion of good and bad cholesterol.) This disorder is called familial hypercholesterolemia, or FH, and occurs in about one in every 400 individuals. FH responds to a diet low in saturated fat and cholesterol (see Chapter 11) but most often requires the addition of cholesterol-lowering medications for its control. Fortunately there are now many such medications and new ones are being discovered.

The second most common inherited problem is now known as insulin resistance, or IR, a disorder in which the body resists the action of insulin in removing glucose from the blood. Those with IR are susceptible to later-developing Type 2 diabetes, especially given the weight gain and decrease in exercise that usually occurs in adulthood. The simplest clue to the presence of IR is a high blood triglyceride level (over about 200). Avoiding weight gain, maintaining good exercise levels, and decreasing consumption of refined sugars and convenience foods made with white flour can do a great deal to counter IR, and even make it undetectable. (For further discussion, see Chapters 3, 10, and 11.)

A genetic predisposition to a high level of homocysteine, an amino acid that favors plaque formation and increases the tendency of the blood to clot, can also be inherited.

Keep in mind that people with inherited risk factors can do a great deal to avoid heart attacks and live longer if they improve their risk profile through lifestyle changes.

3

Risk and Protective Factors for Heart Disease

Risk factors are behavioral patterns or physical characteristics that increase the risk of developing a particular disease—in this case, heart disease. On the other hand, there are behaviors and conditions that decrease your risk, known as *protective factors*. The goal is to reduce your risk of heart disease by minimizing or eliminating the risk factors and by taking advantage of protective factors. Those who already have heart disease can use this same formula to help retard the progress of the disease and, in some cases, even reverse it.

Both risk and protective factors can be divided into two groups: *lifestyle factors*, that is, factors you can control by changing your behavior, such as modifying your diet, avoiding harmful environmental influences, or taking medication; and *innate factors* out of your control, such as genetic traits (which can either be protective or cause increased risk) and previous illnesses. While it is necessary for you to become familiar with the latter group, the innate factors, in order to fully understand your heart disease (or risk of heart disease), it is your control over the first group, the lifestyle factors, that allows you to fully participate in your treatment and recovery. It is the intent of this book to assist you in learning about controllable risk and protective factors and to guide you in *responsibly making whatever changes you can to minimize or reverse heart disease or the risk of heart disease*.

WHAT ARE THE RISK FACTORS FOR HEART DISEASE?

The risk factors for heart disease include

Lifestyle Risk Factors

- smoking
- high blood cholesterol
- high LDL cholesterol ("bad" cholesterol)
- low HDL cholesterol ("good" cholesterol)
- high blood triglycerides (a type of blood fat)
- high blood pressure
- diabetes
- high blood homocysteine (an amino acid that increases the blood's tendency to clot)
- use of oral contraceptives
- being overweight or obese
- physical inactivity
- stress (especially anger and hostility)
- depression
- lack of social support
- poor diet

Innate Risk Factors

- family history of heart disease
- personal history of heart disease
- age (the older you are, the higher the risk)
- gender (males and postmenopausal women at higher risk)
- high blood cholesterol
- high LDL cholesterol ("bad" cholesterol)
- low HDL cholesterol ("good" cholesterol)
- high blood triglycerides (a type of blood fat)

How do I figure out my risk profile?

If you have been diagnosed with heart disease, you probably already know if you have high blood pressure, high blood cholesterol, or diabetes. Some risk factors, like smoking, being overweight, or having a sedentary lifestyle, do not need to be diagnosed by someone else—you can diagnose them yourself. To assess other risk factors, such as high blood pressure or high blood cholesterol, you need to undergo medical tests. If you have heart disease, high cholesterol, or diabetes, it is likely that your health care professionals have gone over your heart disease risk profile with you; if not, be sure to request this service. You can begin with this self-scoring chart.

SIMPLIFIED SELF-SCORING TEST OF CHRONIC DISEASE RISK

Risk habit or factor	Increasing risk				
Smoking cigarettes	None	Up to 9 per day	10 to 24 per day	25 to 34 per day	35 or more per day
Score	0	1	2	3	4
Body weight	Ideal weight	Up to 9 lbs. excess	10 to 19 lbs. excess	20 to 29 lbs. excess	30 lbs. or more excess
Score	0	1	2	3	4

Risk habit or factor	Increasing risk				
Blood pressure upper reading (if known)	Less than 110	110 to 129	130 to 139	140 to 149	150 or over
Score	0	1	2	3	4
Blood cholesterol level (if known)	Less than 150	150 to 169	170 to 199	200 to 219	220 or over
Score	0	1	2	3	4
Self-rating of physical activity	Vigorous exercise 4 or more times/week 20 min. each	Vigorous exercise 3 or more times/week 20 min. each	Vigorous exercise 1 to 2 times/week	U.S. average occasional exercise	Below average exercises rarely
or Walking rating	Brisk walking 5 times/week 45 min. each	Brisk walking 3 times/week 30 min. each	Brisk walking 2 times/week 30 min. each	Normal walking 2½ to 4½ miles daily	Normal walking less than 2½ miles daily
Score	0	1	2	3	4
Self-rating of stress and tension	Rarely tense or anxious *or* Yoga, meditation, or equivalent 20 min./day	Calmer than average Feel tense about 3 times/week	U.S. average Feel tense or anxious 2 or 3 times/day Frequent anger or hurried feelings	Quite tense Usually rushed Occasionally take tranquilizer	Extremely tense Take tranquilizer 5 times/week or more
Score	0	1	2	3	4

Note: (1) Subtract 1 point if dietary fiber intake is high (almost all cereals whole grain, almost no sugar, and considerable fruit and vegetable intake). (2) If you are a female taking estrogen or birth control pills, add 1 point if score is 12 or below, 2 points if risk score is 13 or above (especially if you smoke, are overweight, have high blood pressure or high blood cholesterol). (3) Add 1 point for each 10 points of blood pressure above 150 and 1 point for each 30 points of cholesterol above 220. (4) Subtract 1 point if high-density cholesterol level (the protective cholesterol fraction that increases with exercise) is greater than 50.

Enter your total score here _____ .

HOW TO INTERPRET YOUR RESULTS

(Risks are given for cardiovascular disease. These apply, but with less precision, for adult-onset diabetes and diet-related cancers of the breast and colon. For smoking-related cancer of the lungs, the predominant risk is duration and amount of smoking.)

Zone   Score (Maximum points = 24)

F   20–24
The probability of having a premature heart attack or stroke is about four to five times the U.S. average. Action is urgent. Try to drop 4 points within a month and 3 more points within six months.

E   16–19
Incidence of heart attack or stroke is about twice the U.S. average. Action is urgent. Try to drop 4 points within six months and continue reduction.

D   12–15

The U.S. average is 13. This is an uncomfortable and readily avoidable zone. Careful planning can result in a 5- to 6-point reduction within a year.

C   8–11

The likelihood of having a heart attack or stroke is about one half the U.S. average. This is a zone rather easily achieved by most people within a year if they are now in zone D or E. Careful planning can result in a 4- to 6-point reduction within a year.

B   4–7

Incidence of heart attack or stroke about one quarter of the U.S. average. This goal is achievable by many but often takes one or two years to reach.

A   0–3

Incidence of heart attack or stroke rates very low, averaging less than one tenth the rate in the U.S. 35–65 age group. This goal requires diligent effort and considerable family support, and often takes three to four years to reach. Individuals in this range should be proud and gratified (and will often find themselves serving as role models and lending support to the many who have not achieved this very low-risk zone).

What are the most important risk factors in heart disease?

It makes sense that the more risk factors present, the worse the risk. But risk factors are thought to be more than just cumulative; when several are present in your life, it is believed that they can actually *multiply* the risk of heart disease. Research studies are still attempting to quantify the elements of risk. It is very difficult to isolate the value of each risk factor, since people who smoke, for example, often have high blood pressure, too. And people with high blood pressure are often stressed and get little exercise. Fortunately for all of us, protective factors are more than cumulative as well: combine good food choices with exercise and weight control, and their benefits add up to more than the sum of the individual factors.

Trying to rank risk factors can be risky in itself. Doing so can lead to underestimating the importance of any of the single factors. But if we had to choose a couple of risks to put at the top of the list, they would have to be *high blood cholesterol level* and *cigarette smoking*. But high blood pressure and lack of exercise are also among the "top four" risk factors.

What is the risk from cigarette smoking?

Smoking greatly increases your risk of developing heart disease. Depending on the duration of tobacco use, those who smoke up to 25 cigarettes a day are almost twice as likely to develop heart disease as those who don't smoke; those who smoke 25 to 34 cigarettes a day are about three times as likely; and those who smoke more than 35 cigarettes a day are four times as likely to develop heart disease as nonsmokers. There are many ways that smoking contributes to heart disease. Read Chapter 8 if you, or those you care about, smoke.

Why is cholesterol bad for me?

It is a common misconception that cholesterol is some "evil" substance; actually, what's bad is *too much* or *the wrong kind* of cholesterol in the blood. Your body already makes all you need; you do not need to take in extra cholesterol. In fact, in people with normal levels of blood cholesterol, cholesterol taken into the body from food—up to a certain level—just tells the liver to produce a little less. But other food components, like saturated fat, seem to cause the liver to make *more* cholesterol in most people.

Too much cholesterol can lead to arterial clogging—*atherosclerosis*, the condition underlying coronary heart disease. Studies have shown that the higher the total blood cholesterol, the more likely an individual is to develop heart disease. For every 1 percent decrease in the total blood cholesterol of an individual, there is a 2 to 3 percent decrease in heart disease. The higher the blood cholesterol levels in a region or country, the higher the risk of dying of heart disease for residents of that area. This was shown in *The Seven Countries Study* by Dr. Ancel Keys, a classic study published in the 1980s. A graphic representation of this link between blood cholesterol and heart disease is shown in Figure 3-1.

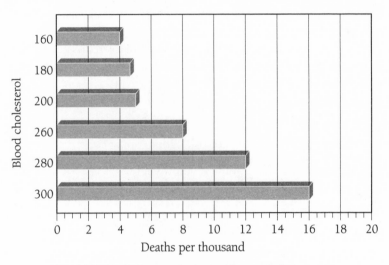

Figure 3-1. Graph showing deaths (per thousand) from coronary
heart disease and cholesterol level

What are "good" cholesterol and "bad" cholesterol?

Blood cholesterol is found in particles called *lipoproteins,* a term
derived from *lipo,* which means fat, and protein. Lipoproteins are
complex particles that float around in the blood and contain more
or less fat and more or less protein, along with cholesterol and a few
other compounds. The more fat they contain, the lighter they are.
Lipoproteins are formed in various organs of the body such as the
intestinal wall and the liver, and as they travel through the blood,
they are modified in various ways. While there are many lipoproteins, we need to focus on only two of them when we think heart
disease: LDL and HDL.

The most common of the light lipoproteins is LDL (low-density
lipoprotein). LDL is often called the "bad" type of cholesterol because it is this type that deposits as plaque in the arteries. High levels of LDL are a major predictor of heart trouble.

The more protein lipoproteins contain, the heavier they are, and
the most common of these is HDL (high-density lipoprotein). The
cholesterol found in HDL has become known as "good" cholesterol.
Not only does it *not* clog arteries, it is protective against heart dis-

ease, apparently because it acts as a "shuttle service" that removes excess cholesterol from tissues, including the arteries, and brings it to the liver. From there it can be made ready for excretion by the body. The word lipoprotein has no meaning when applied to food. You can't say that a food is high or low in HDL or LDL, only high or low in dietary cholesterol, or high or low in fat.

What are healthy levels of cholesterol?

Total blood cholesterol should be below 200 milligrams per deciliter (mg/dl). But it is also important to know your levels of HDL ("good" cholesterol) and LDL ("bad" cholesterol). Any HDL below 35 mg/dl is considered to be abnormal. Women have an average HDL of about 55 mg/dl, and men about 44 mg/dl. Unlike total and LDL cholesterol, for HDL cholesterol, "higher is better and lower is worse" in a sliding scale from between 20 and 70 mg/dl. It is thought that one of the main reasons premenopausal women have a lower heart attack rate than men stems from the protection associated with their having higher HDL levels, most likely due to the presence of estrogen. HDL levels influence risk *independent* of total cholesterol. In other words, even if your total cholesterol is considered "normal," if your HDL is less than 35, then you are still at an increased risk. For those with heart disease, LDL levels below 100 mg/dl are now recommended, but levels up to 130 are considered safe if you don't have other risk factors. As with total cholesterol levels (below 200 mg/dl is considered desirable), there is a sliding scale of risk.

Although some heart disease prevention experts recommend the use of ratios of "bad" to "good" cholesterol, we recommend instead that you *know your numbers* for both good and bad. (See Table 3-1 for these values.) If the good cholesterol is low (your HDL), then work even harder to lower your so-called bad cholesterol.

How do I lower my cholesterol level?

When the control mechanism for cholesterol production in the liver is not able to reduce your blood cholesterol on its own (either because it is malfunctioning or because it has been overwhelmed by too much dietary cholesterol and saturated fat), you must be extra cautious about the foods you eat. Take care to reduce your intake of saturated fats (present mostly in animal fat) since they tend to raise blood cholesterol levels. Smoking, physical inactivity, and stress have also been linked to higher cholesterol levels.

Many drugs that lower cholesterol are effective because they block cholesterol's production by the liver. On the other hand, as you might imagine, since cholesterol is an essential compound for the synthesis of other vital biochemical molecules, these cholesterol-lowering drugs may have some adverse effects in some sensitive people (see Chapter 5 on medications).

What are triglycerides?

Triglycerides are the common fats in the blood. You need them, just as you need cholesterol in your body. Some of the triglycerides are burned by the muscles for energy, while others are stored in fat tissue or circulate in the blood. Some of these free-floating triglycerides can end up lodged in arterial plaque deposits. They are often overlooked as a risk factor, since their relationship to heart disease is not as well documented as that of cholesterol. High intake of refined carbohydrates, too little physical activity, excess weight, a family history of diabetes, and a low fiber intake all conspire to raise the level of these fats in the blood. If your triglycerides tend to be too high, cut down on foods made with white flour and avoid concentrated sugar products (get your sugars from fresh or dried fruits). Replace some high-sugar foods with foods containing the good fats, such as avocado, olive oil, and nuts (see Chapter 11). Excessive alcohol intake can also raise blood triglycerides. If you drink alcoholic beverages, it is best to drink them with meals and in moderation.

Why do some people with high cholesterol still live to a very old age?

While the likelihood of someone with high cholesterol having a heart attack and dying prematurely is much higher than if they had low cholesterol, that doesn't mean everyone with high cholesterol will die prematurely, just as people who smoke two packs of cigarettes a day will not all die of lung cancer. But it is not sensible to simply believe that you will be one of the lucky ones.

Table 3-1. Values for Blood Cholesterol Fractions and Blood
Triglycerides

Total cholesterol
    Desirable—below 200 (below 180 is even better)
LDL cholesterol (the "bad" cholesterol)
    Desirable—below 120 (below 100 if you have heart disease or two
    other risk factors)
    High—above 130
    Very high risk— above 160
HDL cholesterol (the "good" cholesterol)
    High protection—above 50 (high levels are protective)
    Slight protection—between 40 and 50
    Slight risk—between 35 and 40
    High risk—below 35
Triglycerides
    Desirable—below 150 (below 100 is even better)
    Slight risk—between 150 and 200
    High risk—above 200
    Very high risk—above 300

How serious a risk is high blood pressure?

High blood pressure, or hypertension, is one of the four most important heart disease risk factors (along with smoking, high blood cholesterol, and physical inactivity). Hypertension damages the inside
of arteries and increases cholesterol buildup in plaques inside the
artery. Risk of heart attack and stroke rises in a stepwise fashion as
blood pressure goes up from normal levels.

What is blood pressure?

Blood pressure is a measurement of the pressure exerted by the blood
rushing through the arteries. It is controlled mainly by the heart muscle, the many small arteries (arterioles) in the circulatory system, and
proper kidney function. The strength of the heart determines the
force with which the blood is pumped; the size of the small arteries
(and their clear or clogged condition) determines arterial resistance
to blood flow, and the kidneys control the amount of fluids in the
body, which raise or lower the volume of blood.

When blood pressure is taken, two sets of numbers are recorded: the higher number is the systolic pressure, measured at the peak of the heart's contraction (from the Greek *systellein*, "to shorten"), and the lower number is the diastolic pressure, measured when the heart is dilated and resting for an instant between beats (from the Greek *diastellein*, "to dilate"). The *normal* range, when you are resting and free from stress, varies somewhat but should be lower than 130 for systolic pressure and less than 85 for diastolic pressure. When the blood pressure readings on repeated tests are above 140 systolic and 90 diastolic (written as 140/90), most doctors will diagnose you as having hypertension. When the reading is greater than 160/90, the nurse or doctor will start to frown and set a treatment plan in motion, often recommending one of the many blood-pressure-lowering medications. Such a high reading should also be a signal to work very hard on lifestyle (protective) factors. It's normal for blood pressure to rise during physical activity, but it should return to normal soon after the end of your exercise. It can also rise because of stress or anxiety. For example, the stress induced by a visit to a physician's office can result in a false high blood pressure reading, which in medical jargon is called *white-coat hypertension*. Before blood pressure is measured, always rest for a while and relax, and get more than one measurement.

How does high blood pressure affect my heart?

There are two primary ways high blood pressure can damage the heart. One is by increasing deposits of cholesterol in the coronary arteries, which happens because the extra pressure damages the inner lining of the arteries. Scientists have labeled the origin of this damage "shear stress," akin to the pitting and deposits of calcium seen in water pipes in areas of greater turbulence, such as when a smaller pipe is joined to a larger pipe. High blood pressure can also affect the heart muscle itself. Hypertension occurs because the thousands of small arteries in the body are slightly narrowed, making it necessary for the heart muscle to push blood through greater *resistance*. The greater the resistance, the higher the pressure needed, and the higher the blood pressure that is measured at the arm. After some years of this extra workload, the heart muscle gets thicker; this is called *left ventricular hypertrophy*. The process is very similar to the muscle enlargement that occurs in a weight lifter—thus one could say that the heart is lifting an extra weight every time it has to beat against the extra resistance caused by narrowing of the body's many small arteries. If the heart has to make this extra pumping effort for many years, heart failure can result due to pure overwork, rather than to heart attacks caused by plaque-laden arteries.

What can I do to lower my blood pressure?

While the cause of high blood pressure is difficult to pinpoint, there are ways it can be lowered through changes in behavior. Here are some ways that have been shown to help lower blood pressure in people with hypertension:

- giving up cigarette smoking (see Chapter 7)
- controlling stress (see Chapter 8)
- getting regular exercise (see Chapter 9)
- losing weight if you are overweight or obese (see Chapter 10)
- eating plenty of whole foods low in sodium and high in potassium and calcium, that is, plant foods and nonfat dairy products (see Chapter 11)
- having no more than two drinks per day (one "drink" is one bottle of beer, a glass of wine, or one highball)
- reducing coffee consumption to two cups (or less) per day

You can do a lot yourself to control your blood pressure. You might call this the *natural* way of blood pressure control. If you lower your stress level, change your food choices, lose weight, reduce coffee and alcohol consumption, quit smoking, and increase your physical exercise, and your blood pressure is *still* too high, medication may be required. But with the lifestyle changes we have suggested, even if you need medication, you'll need a lower dose, which will save you money and decrease side effects, complications, and discomfort.

Why is diabetes on the list of risk factors?

Almost 9 million Americans now have diabetes, and there are more than 600,000 new cases every year. About 59,000 Americans died from diabetes in 1995.

The most common type of diabetes, and the kind you can do something about, is called *adult-onset* or *Type 2* diabetes. It usually develops in adulthood, usually doesn't require insulin for its treatment, and is diagnosed when your morning blood sugar is over about 120 mg/dl. Being overweight is one of the major predisposing factors of Type 2 diabetes. Weight loss, especially if it is accompanied by increased exercise, often reverses many of the health problems associated with this type of diabetes, and may return you to a completely normal blood sugar level. (At this point you no longer have the diabetes diagnosis, but you are susceptible to it, and it will return if you regain the weight.) High blood pressure, which often goes together with Type 2 diabetes, usually returns to normal with weight loss.

Diabetes causes heart disease through three main mechanisms. First, the high blood pressure that accompanies diabetes will harm the arteries as described above. Second, a diabetic is usually at higher risk from elevated blood triglyceride levels (over 200) and from lower levels of HDL (below 35), the protective fraction of cholesterol. These two risk factors of blood lipids increase deposits of cholesterol in the heart arteries. The third risk factor is the high blood sugar itself: it isn't understood why this occurs, but as blood sugar rises, the amount of cholesterol deposited in the arteries increases.

Whatever you do, *don't let your diabetes go untreated!* This is a wake-up call to lose weight, to increase exercise, to lower your sugar intake, and to work *harder* to lower any of your risk factors (by lowering blood pressure, triglycerides, and LDL; by increasing your HDL and your exercise levels). Exercise alone will lower blood triglycerides and raise HDL (these two occur together), and of course it will aid in weight loss and will help lower blood pressure. Exercise helps diabetics, even if no weight is lost, by increasing our muscles' ability to take sugar out of the bloodstream. Weight loss itself, when achieved by diet alone, also lowers blood sugar, so the combination has a double benefit. If weight loss, increased exercise, and lowered sugar intake do not make your diabetes disappear, you must see your doctor and get one of the many medications now available to lower blood sugar. With a severe case of diabetes (in those with a strong genetic susceptibility), progression of the diabetes over time may eventually lead to a need for insulin injections. But the more you improve your lifestyle, the less likely it is that this will be needed.

I've never heard of homocysteine. Is it a serious risk factor?

While some research as far back as 1968 showed that homocysteine was a risk factor, it was only recently that we found out the major role it may play in heart disease. Homocysteine is one of the many amino acids (the building blocks of our bodies' proteins) found in the blood. Many clinical laboratories are now measuring it. Higher levels of homocysteine cause heart disease by increasing the tendency of blood to clot and by damaging the walls of the arteries, which favors cholesterol deposits. It was thought that normal levels of homocysteine were between 5 and 12 micromoles per liter, but new evidence points out that you should be concerned when your level is over 9 micromoles per liter. Moreover, it appears that an increase in your blood homocysteine level of even a few units increases your risk of heart disease: a 5 unit increase could be as bad as a 30 milligram increase in blood cholesterol.

Although high levels of homocysteine are found in people with the rare genetic disorder homocystinuria, they more commonly occur in people whose diets are low in folic acid (a vitamin in the B-complex group) and also low in vitamins B_6 and B_{12}. Other factors that increase homocysteine levels in the blood are a diet high in animal protein, smoking, heavy consumption of unfiltered coffee, stress, estrogen deficiency, and low thyroid hormone.

In addition to increasing the risk of heart disease, high homocysteine levels have been linked to increased risk for dementia (such as Alzheimer's disease), to the deterioration of eyesight with aging, to stroke, to hypertension, and to various problems in pregnancy and lactation such as premature delivery, low birth weight, early miscarriage, and neural tube defects.

How can I lower my homocysteine level?

Eating lots of legumes (especially lentils), whole grains, fruits, and vegetables (particularly those with green leaves—see Chapter 11) helps homocysteine levels return to normal. As B vitamins are soluble in water, it is best to steam or microwave vegetables with little or no water. Despite a healthy diet with an adequate amount of folic acid, some individuals may need supplemental amounts. Some easy steps to help lower your homocysteine level are: take a good multivitamin supplement that contains folic acid, B_6, and B_{12}; decrease meat and other animal protein intake, or eliminate meat altogether if your homocysteine level is very high; find some time every day for meditation to relieve stress; limit alcohol intake; avoid drinking strong coffee; and exercise more. And do not smoke.

Remember that the steps that help lower homocysteine levels are the same that help reduce other heart disease risk factors.

I hear women have less risk of heart disease than men. Is this true?

The rate of heart disease in premenopausal women is approximately half that of men. However, following menopause women catch up to men within ten years and even have slightly higher rates after age seventy. The problem is that heart disease in women often goes undiagnosed in both younger and older women. The reason for this underdiagnosis stems from two sources: society in general, including women, has developed a false sense of security, believing that women are protected; and physicians and other health care professionals have habitually underestimated the extent of heart disease in women, although recent publicity has partly remedied this situation. Greater attention and publicity must be given to this problem.

What risks are associated with oral contraceptives?

Oral contraceptives pose a risk for heart disease because they raise slightly the level of LDL cholesterol while at the same time lowering the level of HDL. However, among nonsmoking women under forty who take birth control pills, there is only a slight increase in the risk of heart disease. But when women in the same age group smoke, are overweight, *and* take birth control pills, they are about five times more likely to suffer a heart attack.

What about being overweight?

First we need to clearly define what it is to be overweight. Most women not only are aware of their weight status but are actually likely to overestimate how overweight they are; men have the opposite problem. The simplest way of determining your ideal weight is to do the "pinch test." Pull out on the skin at your waist just above your hip. If it is less than an inch and close to the width of your little finger, you are the unusual person who is at his or her ideal weight. It has been found that excess weight at the waistline is more damaging than excess weight on the hips or arms—this is the so-called male pattern of obesity, because men are more likely to put on extra weight at the waistline.

We also recommend a formula adapted from those used in a previous book by one of the authors: *The American Way of Life Need Not Be Hazardous to Your Health* (by John Farquhar). For men, ideal weight equals height in inches times 4 minus 120; for women, height in inches times 3.5 minus 100. Thus for a 5-foot-5-inch woman, ideal weight is 127.5 pounds. For most of us, excess weight does not increase heart disease risk until you are about 10 or 15 percent above your ideal, and generally after that point the risk increases as your degree of overweight increases.

Being overweight doesn't carry the same risk for everyone. For those with a family history of Type 2 diabetes, as little a weight gain as 5 percent over what is called "ideal" body weight increases the risk of heart disease. These individuals develop insulin resistance and high blood triglyceride levels, the precursors of this type of diabetes.

Carrying excess weight has been shown to increase total cholesterol and especially triglycerides, while lowering the good HDL cholesterol. Being overweight is one of the biggest triggers of high blood pressure, a prime contributor to heart disease. If we look at all the factors affecting high blood pressure, weight loss appears to be the single most effective means of lowering it. Also, as described earlier, losing extra weight, especially when combined with increased exercise, can have a profound effect on diabetes, even to the point of leading to a normal blood sugar level, as well as important lowering of blood triglycerides. Read Chapter 10 for a more thorough discussion of weight and heart disease, and Chapter 11 to learn about good food choices for a healthy heart.

Just how important is physical activity?

Pretty important. We know that people who do not get regular exercise have about twice as many heart attacks as people who do. They also have higher cholesterol and triglyceride levels, higher blood pressure, and more excess weight than those who get regular aerobic exercise. No matter what the degree of overweight, sedentary people are more likely to develop Type 2 diabetes, and in a more severe form—that is, their blood sugars will be higher. See Chapter 10 for more information on physical activity and guidelines for starting an exercise program.

Can stress really damage the heart?

It certainly can, and by many different mechanisms. Stress that isn't handled well, especially if accompanied by bouts of anger, can increase the outpouring of the stress hormones, such as cortisol, adrenaline, and noradrenaline, all from the adrenal gland—the small powerhouse gland that sits on top of our kidneys. Stress hormones can do the following:

- increase pulse rate and blood pressure
- push up triglyceride levels
- increase the clotting tendency of our blood
- increase the chances of rupturing one of the plaques, which can be a cause of an acute heart attack
- cause an arrhythmia (an abnormal rapid heartbeat), which can also trigger a heart attack.

Are depression and loneliness bad for your heart?

In those who have survived one heart attack, the chances of survivors with depression having a second heart attack within the next two years is double that of nondepressed survivors. Poor coping with stress can be one of the many causes of depression. Lack of social support, such as a comforting spouse or friends, has been shown to lead to increased stress and depression, and to a lower survival rate after a heart attack. We therefore discuss the social support issue in the section on stress. Keep in mind that if social support can help a heart attack survivor, it can also help prevent the first one from occurring.

What are the most important protective factors?

Some key protective factors you have under your control are

- weight control (see above)
- avoiding tobacco use and secondhand smoke (see Chapter 8)
- relaxation or meditation (see Chapter 9)
- dealing with stress, depression, and lack of social support (see Chapter 9)
- physical activity (see Chapter 10)
- proper food choices (see Chapter 11)
- genetic factors (see below)

Most of these, like the lifestyle risk factors, are linked to your way of life. However, some protective factors are inherited. Just as there are genetic causes of high LDL levels, there are families with a history of longevity who inherit *low* cholesterol and LDL levels. Longevity has also been reported in families with *high* levels of HDL, the protective fraction of cholesterol. There is considerable evidence from studies of identical twins reared apart to show that the degree of overweight has a strong genetic basis. This also means that the important protective factor of remaining close to one's ideal body weight has a fairly strong genetic component. In a similar vein, just as hypertension has a genetic component, so does the protective factor of having a blood pressure that is below the average for the population at large. For those who have inherited protective factors, it is still important to avoid tobacco and a sedentary lifestyle. For those who inherit a susceptibility to the risk factors of cholesterol, triglycerides, blood pressure, body weight, and Type 2 diabetes, it is even more important to adopt and maintain diet, exercise, and stress management routines in order to decrease the inherited risk tendency.

Think about your personal risk profile and focus first on the chapters that discuss the risk factors that apply to you. The best news is that you will find that the same corrective behaviors work to reduce or eliminate many different risk factors, and you may actually find it an enjoyable challenge to learn about these tools in the chapters that follow. When heart disease is advanced, or when the marvelous benefits of food and exercise, weight control, smoking cessation, and control of stress and depression are not sufficient, other means such as medications and surgery may be necessary.

4

Diagnostic Tests

There are many tests that can show your physician the condition of your heart and, if you are recovering from a heart attack, how well you are doing now. These tests range from a routine blood test in a doctor's office and other noninvasive procedures to complex tests, some requiring a hospital session.

What are invasive and noninvasive procedures?

In noninvasive procedures, nothing penetrates your body except perhaps a needle to draw some blood from your arm. A good example is an electrocardiogram, in which electrodes are attached to the outside of your chest. Sometimes when your physcian suspects a major problem and you could be a candidate for surgery, an invasive procedure can give better and more reliable information than the noninvasive type. A good example of an invasive procedure is when a catheter—a flexible, fine plastic tube—is inserted through a blood vessel in the arm or leg. The physician pushes this flexible tube into the heart, most often to inject dye for an angiogram to find out where the blockages are in the heart's arteries (the *coronary* arteries).

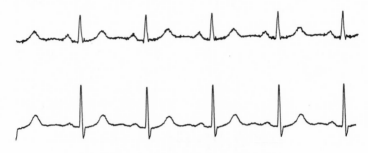

Figure 4-1. Electrocardiogram tracing

What is an electrocardiogram?

An electrocardiogram, or ECG (E = electro, C = cardio or heart, G = gram as in writing—think of grammar), measures the electrical activity of the heart. Electrodes are attached to your chest, wrists, and ankles, and the electrical signals they measure are recorded on paper or on a computer screen. Abnormalities in the pattern of waves can be interpreted by your physician as possible signs of heart disease.

The most common type of ECG is called a *resting* ECG, because it is performed while you are lying down. This test is often part of a routine physical exam, but is *not* very revealing unless you have major damage to your heart. Much more revealing is the *exercise* ECG, done while you walk or run on a treadmill with the electrodes attached to your chest. This is also called a *stress* ECG, as it tests your heart during the stress of physical activity. A stress ECG reveals damage to the heart caused by a narrowing of the arteries, which prevents sufficient oxygen from getting to the heart muscle: the heart cries out for more oxygen during exercise.

Is the exercise ECG what some people call a treadmill test?

Yes, because you exercise on a treadmill. Years ago, before treadmills came into common use, physicians used a step test with three wooden steps and you walked up and down these steps for a certain amount of time with the electrodes attached to your body.

What are other noninvasive tests?

Some common ones, but not as common as the ECG, include the thallium test, Doppler ultrasonography, the MRI (magnetic resonance imaging), the echocardiogram, and the rarely used chest X ray. All of these tests are generally done in a large clinic or in the outpatient department of a hospital.

In the thallium test, a nonharmful, low-level radioactive metal (thallium) is injected into a vein. The heart is then scanned by a device that shows light spots in parts of the heart that have good blood flow. Dark areas (or cold spots) indicate parts of the heart that are not getting enough blood, which is a sign of previous damage to that region of the heart due to blockage of one of the coronary arteries.

Doppler ultrasonography uses sound waves that create electrical impulses that are visible on a screen. It is mainly used now to look for narrowing due to atherosclerosis in the main arteries of the neck (the carotid arteries) that bring blood to the head.

The MRI uses radio waves to produce a detailed outline of the heart, the heart's chambers and the heart valves. It can be very useful in the diagnosis of heart disease, congestive heart failure, valvular disease, some types of congenital heart disease, and other heart problems. The MRI usually takes about thirty minutes.

The echocardiogram, sometimes just called an "echo," displays sound reflections from structures in the heart and is commonly used to determine how well the heart is functioning. A "stress echo," like the stress electrocardiogram, can reveal problems with heart function by showing the parts of the heart that have suffered damage, for example, from a previous heart attack.

A chest X ray shows a shadow of your heart and lungs. This is valuable only for specific situations such as an enlarged heart and it is a test that is very seldom used. In most cases chest X rays give little information on common forms of heart disease.

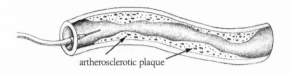

artherosclerotic plaque

Figure 4-2. Catheter in coronary artery for angiogram

Are there blood tests that can help my physician to determine how I am doing?

Yes. During a heart attack, some heart muscle cells that lack sufficient blood and oxygen become damaged, releasing various enzymes
into the bloodstream. A blood sample may be drawn every few hours
to look for these enzymes as one way to diagnose whether a heart
attack has occurred and how much muscle has been damaged.

After a heart attack, your physician will always take blood sam-
ples to measure blood cholesterol and fractions of blood cholesterol.
These tests can reveal your level of risk of developing a future heart
attack (see Chapter 3). These fractions include measures of high-
density lipoprotein cholesterol (HDL), often called the "good" cholesterol, and low-density lipoprotein cholesterol (LDL), often called
the "bad" cholesterol (see page 26). Levels of triglycerides (a type of
fat in the blood) are often measured at the same time.

A friend of mine was tested for Lp(a). What is that?

This is a relatively new blood test. Lp(a), which stands for "lipoprotein small a," is a material produced by the liver that increases the
tendency of the blood to clot. A higher Lp(a) level increases the
risk of a heart attack. It is primarily determined by inheritance and
usually can't be raised or lowered through diet or by most medicines. Premenopausal women have lower levels of Lp(a) than postmenopausal women, because of the presence of circulating estrogen.
If your Lp(a) level is elevated, your doctor will take that into consid-
eration and work harder to lower your other risk factors.

Are there any other blood tests that determine my risk?

Yes, blood homocysteine is now being measured more commonly
(see page 33). Like blood cholesterol, your homocysteine level is a

measure of your risk rather than of heart disease. Homocysteine levels are determined both by genetics and diet (see page 33). Homocysteine and cholesterol testing are important in heart disease prevention and, if you already have heart disease, in the prevention of a second heart attack over the long term.

What is an angiogram?

An angiogram, also called coronary angiography, is based on "cardiac catheterization," which refers to the insertion of a catheter—a small flexible tube—into the heart. This invasive procedure is performed in a hospital. The tube is inserted under local anesthesia through an artery in the arm or groin area of the leg and carefully guided into the heart. After the catheter has reached the heart, a dye is injected that allows the heart's arteries to be measured for narrowing due to atherosclerosis. This procedure is considered the most definitive way to determine how much atherosclerosis you have and is regarded by many cardiologists as the mainstay of heart disease diagnosis.

When an angiogram is done, the doctor might find the narrowing so serious that the catheter is then immediately used as a tool to open the clogged artery seen in the angiogram. This procedure, called angioplasty or balloon angioplasty, is done by inflating a balloon in the artery to squeeze the plaque to a smaller size (see Chapter 6).

5

Medications for Heart Disease

When lifestyle changes are not sufficient to treat your heart disease, many drugs are available. While you should not use drugs to avoid lifestyle changes, often drugs have a place in heart disease management and can save lives. In ancient times, fresh or dried herbs or herbal extracts were the main sources of medicines. Today, the pharmaceutical industry is developing new medications to an extraordinary degree. Some drugs are for short-term use, others may be needed for the rest of your life.

What can heart drugs do for me?

Drugs can lower blood cholesterol and blood pressure and can decrease the tendency of blood to make abnormal clots. Drugs can extend your healthy years and, in certain situations, be lifesaving.

The major types of drugs used in heart disease include

- drugs to lower blood cholesterol or triglycerides
- drugs to control angina
- drugs to control blood pressure
- drugs to control blood clotting
- drugs to control heart rhythm and prevent arrhythmias

If drugs are so effective, why should I change my lifestyle?

We live in a time when people too often think of drugs as magical, relieving us of the need to change our lifestyle choices. For people with heart disease, can today's drugs allow one to avoid lifestyle changes? The answer is, without any doubt, *no*. Lifestyle changes must come in tandem with any drugs your doctor prescribes; drugs should *never* be used in place of lifestyle modification. Many doctors will first advise lifestyle changes for reducing cholesterol levels or other conditions and only prescribe medicine if they fail—but the lifestyle changes, even if minor, should be continued. Lifestyle and medications work together very well.

You must tell your physician that you are willing to give a new lifestyle, from diet to exercise to not smoking (if you are a smoker), a good try. Remember, some people prefer taking a drug to making changes in their routine: *make it clear you are not one of them*.

Look ahead to the chapters on food and weight control, stress, and exercise. Make a concerted effort to keep your weight down and change your meals to those low in animal products and high in whole grains and cereals, vegetables, fruits, legumes, nuts, and other seeds. The more you do in the area of lifestyle changes, the lower the dose of any drug you may need to take, and therefore the less likely you will be to suffer side effects. And better yet, sometimes you may not need any drugs at all.

What about adverse effects of drugs?

This is a time when some great drugs are available, but this is also a time for caution. You should never forget that drugs that are effective are, and have to be, extremely powerful—often they save lives—but that they sometimes have undesirable effects, known as *adverse drug reactions* (ADR) or *side effects*. When it comes to drugs for heart disease, you need to be very candid with your physician. Make her or him aware that you know the *two sides of drug action*. Discuss the adverse effects of any drug prescribed.

If you are on medication and notice any of the adverse effects described in this chapter or that you have been told to watch for by a health professional, contact your physician as soon as possible. Some adverse effects can occur soon after you have started on your new medication—perhaps an upset stomach or signs of your liver undergoing some minor damage. Your physician can uncover possible liver problems by doing a simple blood test. Other more insidious, but fortunately rarer, side effects are long-term. Examples include an increased risk for some cancers.

What about other drugs I am taking?

Many people take more than one prescription drug and often some nonprescription, over-the-counter (OTC) medications and perhaps herbal remedies as well. Keep a list of all the medications you are taking and their doses. Bring this list with you to all doctor visits. Be sure to tell your physician of any other drugs, including vitamins, minerals, and other dietary supplements, and herbs, that you take regularly or that you feel you need to take occasionally. Many drugs interact with each other, and this can lead to adverse effects or some loss of the efficacy of your medication. Entire books have been published on drug interactions. If you go to different specialists for various problems, make all of them aware of the other medications you are taking. The problem of conflicting prescriptions in the complex world of modern managed care is a significant one, and your physician cannot help you unless you keep her or him informed.

What are some types of cholesterol- or triglyceride-lowering drugs?

The most advertised and prescribed cholesterol-lowering drugs today belong to a group of drugs called *statins*. Next come some special resins: *niacin* (nicotinic acid), one of the B vitamins taken in very large amounts; bile-acid-binding *resins;* and the *fibrates*, which are used mostly to lower triglycerides. The key goal of these medications is to lower the LDL (bad) cholesterol, while not lowering the HDL (good) cholesterol, or to lower triglycerides (fat in the blood).

What are the most common cholesterol-lowering drugs prescribed today?

Statins are definitely the most common. The major drug companies are all competing to come out with new statins under various trade names (such as Mevacor, Zocor, and Lipitor), as these are now widely prescribed drugs. They vary in price, and different health maintenance organizations (HMOs) often bargain and sign a contract with a particular drug company, so your physician might say, "I prefer you take this one and not the other one." Each differs in some way in its chemical structure, but all produce the same effect, and in low doses they seem to be quite safe.

How do statins work?

Understanding how statins work will help you understand their possible adverse effects. Statins interfere with the production of cholesterol in the body, mainly in the liver. Since you synthesize your own cholesterol (see Chapter 3), it makes sense to limit the amount you consume if you are an overproducer. The liver—together with cholesterol from food—is responsible for most of the cholesterol found in the blood. There is a key step in cholesterol synthesis that these statins block quite effectively. The result is a reduction in blood LDL cholesterol levels of 25 percent to 45 percent, depending on the dose prescribed.

Since cholesterol is the key molecule for the production—or synthesis—of other essential compounds (like some hormones and bile acids needed for the digestion of fats) in the body, if the dose of the statin is too high there may be some adverse effects.

Always remember: do as much as possible in terms of diet, not smoking, physical activity, and stress management so that if you still need a statin—or any other cholesterol-lowering drug—a low dose will be effective.

What are some of the adverse effects of statins?

Below are the most common possible side effects found in advertisements for various statins. This list is not complete. As with any drug, be sure to ask your physician about side effects before taking statins, read the material that comes with the prescription, and discuss immediately any side effects that occur while you are taking them. On the bright side, these side effects usually affect only 2 to 4 percent of people taking statins.

Some common adverse effects of statins are

- muscle tenderness or weakness
- unexplained muscle aches
- allergic reactions
- liver function abnormalities
- insomnia
- skin rash and itching
- headache
- indigestion
- loss of appetite (anorexia)

There are other possible side effects, but their occurrence is extremely rare.

Which common drugs might the statins interact with adversely?

Some of the statins may interact adversely with niacin (nicotinic acid), erythromycin, drugs that fight fungal infections, and drugs that suppress the immune system (immunosuppressive drugs), and may increase the potency of some anti-blood-clotting drugs (anticoagulants) based on warfarin.

If you have more than one physician, let each physician know of the other medications and herbal supplements you are taking.

Can I use a statin if I am pregnant?

Statins are *not* to be used during pregnancy—they may cause damage to the fetus—or by nursing mothers. If you are a woman of childbearing age, you should only use statins if you definitely do not plan to become pregnant. The general rule in medicine today is that only in situations of extremely high blood cholesterol that do not respond to nondrug treatments like diet should statins be given to women of childbearing age.

What is niacin, a drug or a vitamin?

Niacin is nicotinic acid, one of the B vitamins. It's found in many foods, especially whole grains and milk products. As a vitamin, you need only about 15 milligrams of niacin a day. However, when used to lower cholesterol niacin is used in what are called *pharmacological* levels rather than in vitamin amounts. One positive side to niacin is that it's the least expensive of all cholesterol-lowering medications available, although the drug does have a high rate of side effects.

The pharmacological levels can range from a few hundred up to 6,000 milligrams per day. If you take 100 milligrams, the only side effect you may experience is some flushing and warmth for a few minutes (this dosage is too low to lower blood cholesterol). When you are taking 1,000 to 6,000 milligrams a day, the rate of side effects is very high. The minimum dose for any real effect on cholesterol is about 1,000 milligrams. One usually starts with 100 milligrams (or a few hundred milligrams), slowly increasing the dose to over 1,000 milligrams. Only about two out of three people can tolerate the required dose. The most common complaints are indigestion and flushing. Some special formulations are becoming available that are absorbed more slowly and appear to cause less flushing and fewer side effects.

Niacin can raise blood sugar levels, so if you have diabetes, niacin should not be taken. Niacin is one of the few drugs that can lower triglycerides as well as cholesterol, and that, together with the very low price, is why it is still prescribed. Nationally, the number of prescriptions written annually for niacin is very low, but that figure is misleading because niacin is available over the counter and could be used for lowering cholesterol without a prescription.

What about resins for lowering cholesterol?

Resins to lower blood cholesterol have been around for a while and they work in a different way than statins. Resins bind bile acids in the intestine, taking them out of your system. What has this to do with cholesterol? Cholesterol is used in the liver to make bile acids. By removing bile acids from your system, you force the liver to use additional cholesterol to make more bile acids, lowering the level of cholesterol in your blood.

While resins are rather effective in small doses, they have lost popularity because of their side effects: indigestion and constipation. Many physicians who run heart clinics recommend them, but many privately practicing physicians who don't prescribe resins as frequently are less likely to recommend them. The advantage of the resins is that they are not absorbed by the body and cannot have any damaging long-term side effects. If you have to take a statin or other drug to lower cholesterol, resins will allow you to use a smaller amount of that drug, which is absorbed into the body and can have some more extensive side effects. Two resins available are cholestyramine and colestipol. Keep in mind their main adverse effects: constipation and indigestion.

There is a wide range of compounds in nature that do something similar to these resins: certain forms of vegetable and fruit fiber, known as *soluble dietary fiber.*

Are you saying that I can find fiber in foods to help lower cholesterol?

Yes. Soluble dietary fibers act in a way similar to resins. You can find these fibers only in foods from plants, which is why heavy consumption of vegetables, whole fruits, beans, grains, nuts, and other seeds is recommended (see Chapter 11). This is one reason for the old saying "An apple a day keeps the doctor away." Soluble dietary fiber binds bile acid, but less aggressively than resins, perhaps one fourth as strongly. If your diet includes a lot of soluble fiber, it will help lower your cholesterol. If you still need bile-acid-binding agents, that dosage will be lower than would otherwise be needed. So, again, food is the mainstay.

Are there fiber supplements I can buy without a prescription?

There are some products on the market that contain psyllium, pectin—a major fiber in fruits and vegetables—and guar gum, or other concentrated soluble fiber. Oat bran contains a cholesterol-lowering fiber that you can find in oatmeal and other whole oat products. Jams and jellies contain pectins from the fruit itself and some added as a jelling agent. There is no doubt that a good soluble fiber supplement can help and, for some people, may be all you need in combination with lifestyle changes.

What are fibrates?

Another class of drugs is called fibrates, and the one most commonly used in the United States has been gemfibrozil. Fenofibrate is another fibrate that has just begun to be used here. Physicians use these two drugs to help lower triglycerides, and fenofibrate also is effective in lowering LDL. Physicians tend to prescribe fibrates for people with high triglycerides as the first line of treatment, although, as we've already said, niacin will also lower triglycerides. It's important to note that the natural way of lowering triglycerides is to use only a moderate amount of alcohol, exercise regularly, stay close to your ideal weight, and eat a diet rich in vegetables and grains and other foods that are very low in sugar. Replacing some breads, potatoes, rice, and corn with soy, seeds, nuts, avocado, and olive oil may aid in lowering triglycerides. This involves a partial replacement of carbohydrate-rich foods with so-called good fats.

Do the fibrates have side effects?

The fibrates tend to have a very low rate of side effects and are generally quite well tolerated. Of course, any medication can cause an allergic reaction in some people, and there are allergic reactions to the fibrates. As with almost any cholesterol-lowering drug, indigestion is also a possible side effect.

Are the margarines that are supposed to lower cholesterol really helpful?

Yes, two such margarines (Benecol and Take Control) are now widely available in supermarkets. They contain plant sterols and related compounds that appear to lower LDL cholesterol by about 10 to 15 percent (see Chapter 11 on diet). These products appear to be safe and, in a manner similar to dietary fiber, may allow you to decrease the dose of stronger cholesterol-lowering drugs such as the statins.

Can a combination of these drugs lower my cholesterol even further?

In some cases doctors prescribe two or more drugs at a time. This is called *combination therapy*. Resins or plant fibers and the new margarines are sometimes given with statins, and their addition can produce a further decrease in LDL cholesterol levels of 20 to 25 percent. The further addition of niacin can produce yet another 15 to 20 percent decrease. The sum of these three types of drugs may result in a decrease in LDL cholesterol levels of up to 70 percent. But you should remember that each drug has its own possible array of side effects and these are now all added together. You should be carefully monitored by your health professional for any such adverse effects from the combination of these powerful drugs.

If I take one of these drugs, should I get my liver function checked?

Yes. Your liver has many functions, one of which is to render nontoxic many harmful compounds that enter your system through food or air. When these detoxifying functions become stressed, some liver enzymes reach abnormal levels. Statins, niacin in large amounts, and the fibrates to a lesser extent can lead to abnormal levels of these enzymes, but you might not notice any specific symptoms. A simple blood test to check your liver function is done *before* you begin taking statins and usually twelve weeks after you start taking them or whenever your dose is increased. If you think something is not right with you, call your physician, who may decide to do a blood test for these liver enzymes. However, there is increasing evidence that moderate increases in these liver enzymes from use of cholesterol-lowering drugs does not result in liver damage.

What about blood pressure medications?

The field of blood pressure medication is very complex. There are many classes of compounds, like diuretics, beta-blockers, ACE inhibitors, angiotension receptor blockers (ARBs), calcium-channel blockers, and others. You can ask your physician to describe the effects and side effects of any medication prescribed. The good news is that you can do a great deal to lower blood pressure without drugs, resorting to drugs only for extreme cases or making the needed dose much lower. Again, these drugs have side effects, and if you are taking them, you cannot stop using them abruptly as abnormal surges in blood pressure could cause major trouble, if not death.

Some major side effects of these drugs are as follows:

- all can make the blood pressure fall too low and cause symptoms of faintness and weakness
- diuretics: may cause weakness due to loss of too much of the body's potassium; can raise uric acid, cholesterol, and triglyceride levels, and cause an attack of gout in those who are susceptible to gout
- beta-blockers: most common side effect is weakness and fatigue; can lead to impotence in men, aggravate wheezing in people with asthma, and slightly raise cholesterol and triglyceride levels
- ACE inhibitors: most common side effect is cough; a relatively uncommon side effect is an allergic skin reaction
- angiotension receptor blockers: these are fairly new, can replace ACE inhibitors or any of the other medications, and are relatively free of side effects
- calcium-channel blockers: ankle swelling. Reported benefits are less than those of other blood pressure medications, so use only if others are poorly tolerated

Some of these drugs' actions are easy to understand. A diuretic removes sodium (the part of salt, sodium chloride, that can raise blood pressure), and this decreases the fluid in the bloodstream, thereby decreasing the amount of blood the heart must pump. Beta-blockers decrease the impact of circulating adrenaline by *blocking* its action on the nerves that constrict the small blood vessels, thus making blood flow more easily through these blood vessels.

While medication for blood pressure is sometimes needed, here again, lifestyle changes can play a key role. See Chapters 8 through 11 for ways you can improve your health.

What about blood-clotting medication?

The most important agent to decrease blood clotting is aspirin. It is usually recommended that people who have had a heart attack take either a half or a full aspirin—or what used to be called a baby aspirin—daily to prevent abnormal clumping together of the blood platelets, the small elements in the blood that play a key role in clotting. Clumping is a preliminary step to forming a blood clot, and blood clots can cause problems, including heart attacks, if they form in the coronary arteries.

Treatment with blood-clotting medications other than aspirin, such as warfarin, has to be very carefully supervised by your physician, with blood tests done every few weeks to be sure you are getting the right dose. Major interactions with food can occur with some blood-clotting medications, because some foods—and some vitamin supplements—contain a powerful vitamin, vitamin K, that is part of the blood-clotting mechanism. If you eat more or less of this vitamin, you may need to change the level of your medication. Tell your health professional if you are eating some foods high in vitamin K, like greens—which are very good for you—or taking a supplement containing vitamin K, and that you intend to keep their levels fairly constant.

VITAMIN K-RICH FOODS

- best sources: green leafy vegetables, especially cabbage-family members like broccoli, cabbage, and turnip greens; lettuce; liver
- fortified cereals and meal replacements (like Ensure or Boost)
- smaller amounts: yogurt and other cultured milks, other milk products, other vegetables, fruits, cereals, eggs, and meat

I am postmenopausal; is it true that estrogen is good for my heart?

This is a difficult question to answer, as estrogens have both positive and negative effects in postmenopausal women. Considerable research has suggested that estrogen is protective; however, recent studies have shed doubt on that conclusion, so this remains a controversial issue. There is some concern that prolonged use of estrogen may increase the risk of breast cancer. It is known that estrogen can increase blood triglyceride levels in about 10 percent of susceptible women and this can increase the risk of a heart attack. Women on hormone replacement therapy (HRT) also have an increased blood-clotting tendency. It is important to work with your doctor on this complex question, since the answer is not clear-cut.

Should I keep track of the medications I am taking?

You should write down each of the medicines you're taking and their doses and keep that list with you. Whenever you see any physician, you can show her or him the list to avoid the possibility of any new prescriptions or other recommendations interfering or adversely interacting with any of your current medicines. Your physician, the nurses involved in your care, and the pharmacist who fills your prescriptions should all be able to tell if any drugs you are taking are interacting in the wrong way. It is always a good idea when being prescribed new medicine to ask your doctor to go over the medicines that have already been prescribed for you, along with any herbal products you may take.

6

Major Heart Interventions, from Bypass to Angioplasty

Sometimes invasive intervention or surgery is needed. The coronary arteries may become so narrow that surgery or some other invasive procedure may be the only answer, at least for the present, given the state of our knowledge. Some procedures, even if invasive, are not considered surgery in the classic sense and often are a good way to treat blocked arteries. In medical jargon, physicians talk of *cardiac interventional procedures*. You have the right to discuss these tests with your physician before you decide if you want to have a surgical or other invasive procedure. In this chapter we will focus on procedures for coronary heart diseases, which are by far the most common.

What are the major types of surgery and related procedures?

Surgery ranges from a major procedure where you open the chest surgically and operate on the heart itself—*coronary artery bypass surgery*—to procedures where an instrument is inserted through a blood vessel and threaded through your coronary artery, where it enlarges the narrowed opening, as in *angioplasty*. Even though they are both *invading* your body—that's why they are called *invasive procedures*—the degree of invasion and the related trauma are quite different.

Are there some tests I can have before deciding on surgery or other invasive treatment?

Before a physician decides that you should have bypass surgery or any other kind of invasive treatment, there are various diagnostic procedures that are generally carried out. Two common ones are *electrocardiograms* (ECGs) *on a treadmill* and *angiograms* (see Chapter 4).

What is bypass surgery and when is it recommended?

Bypass surgery is a major surgical operation. The most drastic way to correct the problem of a blocked coronary artery is to replace it with a clean blood vessel from another part of your body. *Replace* is a simplistic term here: what the surgeon actually does is go around the blocked section of the coronary artery by attaching a clean blood vessel—such as a vein from your leg which can be removed without causing problems—to a place just before and to one just after the blockage so the blood can now *bypass* the blocked area and again flow beyond it.

This is not like replacing a clogged pipe in your house with a new, clean one; rather it is like attaching a new pipe to points just before and just after the rusted, blocked region. Just as in your house you would need to turn off the main water valve before putting in the new pipe, so in the case of the heart doctors use special machines to circulate blood and put oxygen into your blood while the heart is being operated on.

What is the outlook for recovery after a bypass?

The outlook is very good. About 500,000 of these operations are performed every year in the United States alone. If, after surgery, the heart attack survivor adopts the right lifestyle and takes medication (if needed), bypasses have a high rate of success.

The rate of failure is very low: about 4 percent of the implanted blood vessels close each year. Failures increase to about 6 percent a year after six years.

If you do not change your lifestyle—continuing smoking being the extreme case—a new bypass may be necessary after a few years. With each successive bypass the rate of success declines. This makes

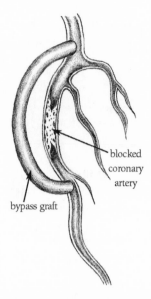

Figure 6-1. Graft bypassing a coronary artery blocked by
atherosclerotic plaque

sense as the heart has already been altered by the first surgery, by a
bypass in place that has failed. The picture gets more and more complex for the surgeon with every operation.

Is angioplasty a surgical procedure?

Angioplasty is not considered a surgical procedure. It is much less
traumatic than a bypass and you should not even think of it as
surgery. Angioplasty is often used as the next step when lifestyle
changes, or lifestyle changes plus medication, do not work. In medical jargon this procedure is referred to as *PTCA*, or *percutaneous transluminal coronary angioplasty.*

A thin tube—catheter—with a balloon tip is inserted after local
anesthesia through a blood vessel in the arm or leg into the blocked
coronary artery. The balloon is repeatedly inflated and deflated to
compress the cholesterol deposit, the plaque, against the wall of the
artery. You may have to stay in the hospital for a day or two. Most of

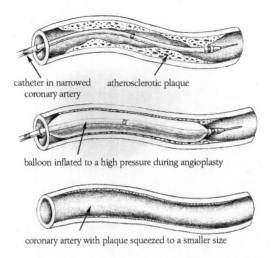

catheter in narrowed   atherosclerotic plaque
coronary artery

balloon inflated to a high pressure during angioplasty

coronary artery with plaque squeezed to a smaller size

Figure 6-2. Catheter in coronary artery before and after angioplasty

the time a coronary artery treated by angioplasty stays open, but in some cases the procedure may need to be repeated after a few months. Again, what you do after this procedure will affect how often, if at all, you need to repeat it.

Sometimes in the midst of an angiogram, if a major blockage in a coronary artery is found, an angioplasty may be performed at the same time while the catheter is already in place.

What are stents?

New advances in the surgical management of coronary artery disease include the growth of the use of *stents*. These are implants made of inert material that are put in an artery to open it up. Stents have had great success in helping people who have very narrowed arteries. Advances are still being made in this area and it's too early to know how successful they will be in the long run. It is important to be treated at a medical center that has had experience with these newer procedures to be sure of getting the best care.

It seems that stents are a step beyond angioplasty; is that correct?

Yes. In angioplasty the coronary arteries are opened, but in 30 to 40 percent of patients, the arteries become narrowed again over time, and ECG exercise treadmill tests show that the blood flow through these arteries is poor. A stent could help prevent a recurrence of this narrowing, which is typical of many angioplasties.

Are there other types of intervention?

There are other procedures that try to clean out the inside of the artery. An example is *atherectomy*. Here, as in angioplasty, a tube is inserted into the narrowed coronary artery. In one type of *atherectomy,* when the tube is in position, a balloon is inflated to hold the tube in place and a blade shaves the plaque from the wall of the artery. The shavings are collected in an attachment and removed when the instrument is taken out.

In a related procedure, a tiny drill attached to a tube is inserted into the problem area. Here the mini-drill grinds the plaque into small pieces that are flushed out by the circulating blood.

Other techniques that are at the forefront of heart surgery include the use of lasers, and studies are in progress to see if special forms of lasers can be used to remove some of the deposits in arteries. With the progress of electronic instrumentation, new techniques are likely to become available.

What are pacemakers?

Pacemakers are miniature lithium-battery-powered devices that take over control of the heartbeat. They are surgically implanted either under the skin or next to the heart and emit electrical impulses. Most commonly, pacemakers are used when the heart beats too slowly due to a disorder called *heart block* (see Chapter 2). Rapid heartbeat disorders called *arrhythmias* may also be treated with pacemakers, but are now more commonly treated through surgical removal of an abnormal electrical pathway in the heart. Many advances in the design of pacemakers and in the surgical control of abnormal heart rhythms have occurred in recent years, including successful miniaturization of pacemakers.

If one of these interventions is recommended, should I get a second opinion?

Having a second opinion is usually a good idea if surgery or an invasive procedure is recommended. Generally physicians are very receptive to such requests and they can recommend a specialist. Don't be afraid to say that you want a second opinion: it's your life and your future. A second opinion may confirm what your personal physician has recommended or may suggest a different option or the possibility of no surgery at all. You can then feel that you have thoroughly weighed the options. *Never forget that the final decision is yours.*

7

Recovery after a Heart Attack

In this chapter you will find the answers to your questions concerning the care you need in the first few weeks after a heart attack. This chapter will be useful not only to heart attack survivors but also to relatives and friends who are helping heart attack survivors readjust to their lives at home.

What are my chances of getting back to my normal life?

The quality of your life after a heart attack will depend on how much of your heart muscle has been injured and the location of the damage: your dietary regimen, medications, and exercise are all determined by the condition of your heart after the heart attack. Many survivors will be able to return to a fully active life as long as they control their risk factors and follow generally accepted disease precautions. For some, the damage may be so extensive that total freedom to live as full a life as before may be unrealistic.

But more and more medical research findings show that most individuals with a heart muscle that has been damaged can resume full activity by the fourth week after the episode, and this includes sexual activity, physical activity, and return to work.

Throughout the entire recovery period, bear in mind the value of the psychological support of a spouse or a close friend.

Will I be an invalid for the rest of my life?

In most cases, as a survivor, you are not an invalid. It is no longer thought that you have to "take it easy" after a heart attack. An early return to work and to full exercise is a new goal in advanced cardiac rehabilitation. This is an important point to keep in mind, and friends and relatives caring for you must recognize this as well. *Invalidism can and must be avoided.* Invalidism has both physical and psychological repercussions, and you will enjoy a fuller recovery if you have confidence that healing is possible and that you can return to a productive life.

There are some exceptional cases that require extra care, and if you are one such case, this would have been discovered during your hospital stay. People who have had major damage to the left ventricle of the heart, the chamber that pumps the blood out into the rest of the body, are at risk for cardiac arrhythmias and may not be able to return to full activity. Your health professional will explain any restrictions that may apply to you. Pay close attention, take notes, and try to have a companion in the room also to write down details. Make sure to ask any and all questions. Your hospital discharge recommendations will make clear whether you should limit your physical activity and exercise; follow the plans outlined very carefully. If you are not one of the exceptional cases, you should enjoy a rather rapid return to regular activity, including sexual activity.

What do I do after I go home?

The first week's home care will depend on the treatments you began in the hospital—for example, whether after your heart attack you received treatment that effectively opened up the blocked arteries preventing blood flow to your heart, or whether you had bypass surgery. And once again, your treatment plan in the first week home depends on the severity of the heart attack. You may be asked to make a return visit to your physician in this first week. *But no matter the severity of your heart attack, it is more important than ever during this first week at home to keep an open lifeline to the hospital and your physician.*

In general, for the first week, expect to take it easy. You may be able to walk on a flat surface at a moderate pace for ten minutes twice a day (morning and afternoon), and you will need to set a new routine. For example, you may wake up, eat breakfast, take a break to do something sedentary, and let your food digest. Then maybe you'll take a shower, relax, take your walk, relax, and have lunch. It will be important to space your activities so that you're not using too much energy, too intensely, all at once. And then evaluate how you feel. Any unusual chest pain, shortness of breath, or irregular or rapid heartbeat should be cause to contact your doctor or the hospital immediately.

What about after the first week?

While in the first week survival is still the key issue in your mind, for the next five weeks or so you should be planning physically, psychologically, and emotionally to return to full activity in your normal life. In this period you have to give it your best effort to achieve full recovery. Focus more than ever on taking your medications, quitting smoking, avoiding secondhand smoke, reducing stress, controlling depression, exercise, and diet, reducing alcohol intake, and lowering your weight if you are obese. The second half of this book is dedicated to discussions of each of these elements of your recovery.

How much influence can I expect to have over my physician?

Sometimes you must impress upon your cardiologist or primary care physician that you are really eager to go beyond standard care, and that you want to go all the way to recovery. Now is the time to be really forceful about expressing your wishes.

Keep in mind that your physician probably has many patients who are not as willing to be aggressive in their approach to reducing their risk factors. You can become an active partner in your care and recovery: ask questions, take notes, learn, ask for copies of your medical records. Do extra reading, even beyond this book. Use the references suggested at the back of this book to gather information that interests you or is specific to your care and recovery. If available, use the Internet to get extra information. Many Web sites now deal with health.

What about cardiac rehabilitation centers?

A cardiac rehabilitation center is a facility located in your community, perhaps at a YMCA or in a hospital. These centers are staffed by nurses trained in the skills needed to supervise physical activity and provide guidance on medications, diet, and rate of recovery after a heart attack. Physicians are readily available if needed and are sometimes in attendance.

These centers can make your recovery much easier and help you build confidence by meeting other people who are recovering successfully from a heart attack. Cardiac rehabilitation centers will help you implement the program outlined in this book, and going to a rehabilitation center can be the very best way to get back to a normal life as soon as possible.

A cardiac rehabilitation program works on all of the risk factors—and your individual program is designed to help you make the transition from knowing in your mind what you need to do to *actually doing it*. You will acquire the skills you need, such as how to check your blood pressure and make sure it is within the guidelines you've been taught and how to exercise at an appropriate level. You will also earn self-assessment skills so you will know what to be concerned about and what is not necessary to report to your physician.

Your initial evaluation at a center gives you an opportunity to have your questions answered and to check your current cholesterol and triglyceride status, your blood pressure, your smoking status, stress factors, and your physical ability to exercise. In addition, you will discuss your current diet, the number of calories you currently take in from fat, and what dietary changes you should make. The evaluation is directed toward getting you to the lowest risk level possible and toward designing the exercise program best for you. Exercise in cardiac rehabilitation is supervised by specialized nurses, with physicians available, too.

Can these centers help with psychological issues, too?

Yes, talking with the health professional at a cardiac rehabilitation center can help you deal with psychological and emotional issues, particularly your fears—fears that can block your progress toward full recovery. Being in a group of others combating their heart disease is sometimes the best psychological boost you can get.

Will the health care system pay for a cardiac rehabilitation program?

Often Medicare covers these programs as long as the Medicare guidelines are met; some HMOs cover these costs, at least for a few months. Some rehabilitation programs are more community-based and try to charge an affordable rate if you want to continue beyond the typical three to four months that are covered by many insurance plans. Call your health plan to see what costs they will cover and for how long.

Where can I find a cardiac rehabilitation program?

Cardiac rehabilitation programs exist throughout the United States, but unfortunately many are underutilized. Only about 30 percent of eligible people actually participate in a cardiac rehabilitation program. After you've found out that you have coronary artery disease, or after you've had a heart bypass or a heart attack, you can significantly decrease your risk of further complications by finding a center nearest you and enrolling in its program. Ask your health care professional or hospital after-care adviser for a referral.

What comes after the end of the first six weeks of recovery?

During the first six weeks, you've been exercising at a lower intensity but steadily increasing the duration of your exercise. At this point, if you leave the rehabilitation program, you should have a clear picture of what heart rate is acceptable and appropriate for you so that your exercise routine doesn't put your heart under strain. By now you should be practically *addicted* to a healthier diet: most people grow to enjoy their new way of eating and slowly, but surely, come to prefer a diet low in animal fats (see Chapter 11).

After week six, you enter what you should consider your *long-term risk factor management* program. Use the second half of this book as your guide to managing your risk factors as part of a normal, healthy lifestyle.

Can a second heart attack be prevented?

In the last five years, research has shown that up to 80 percent of second heart attacks can be prevented. With aggressive risk factor management you can reduce your chance of a second heart attack. This is truly a revolutionary change in expectations. So instead of having a one-in-four chance of a second attack, you now have a one-in-twenty chance. That's really great!

What are the warning signs of a second heart attack?

The signs are the same as for the first: any unexplained chest pain that lasts for more than five minutes. These may occur during exercise, when going out into cold weather, or after a meal. When these pains occur at rest and become more frequent, this is called unstable angina and is a clear signal that a new heart attack might develop. As you have already experienced a heart attack, any pain of this sort and any feeling of pressure or heaviness in the chest are major warning signs. For a heart attack survivor, any of these symptoms require immediate contact with a medical facility or your health care professional.

PART II

THE HEALTHY HEART LIFESTYLE

8

—

Lifestyle Change: Smoking

Almost 28 percent of U.S. men, close to 26 million, and over 23 percent of U.S. women, more than 23 million, smoke today. In addition, about 4,400,000 adolescents between twelve and seventeen years of age smoke.

Most smokers start because of social pressure, because friends smoke, because it appears sophisticated to do so at a party, because it is a forbidden act for the young. (The irony is that most people, when they take their first puff, cough, feel nauseated, and never want to smoke again. Then they force themselves to try again and soon become addicted both physically and psychologically.) An encouraging statistic is that over 40 million Americans are now ex-smokers; the peer pressure that motivated these people to smoke in the first place might just work in reverse now.

If you are a smoker, you will probably have some difficulty reading about the ways in which smoking affects your heart. As you read this information, it may help to keep in mind that the heart disease risk from smoking *is* largely reversible, some of it within the first twenty-four hours after quitting, and the rest of it within three to five years. Also, although you may not like thinking about the specific ways in which smoking causes damage to your heart, having a good picture of how the damage happens may assist you when you decide to quit. A good understanding of the process can help you to visualize the smoothly running cardiovascular system you are working to restore.

How can you say that smoking causes heart disease?

If you ask smokers, nonsmokers, or ex-smokers what they think are the consequences of smoking, no one will hesitate to mention lung cancer, emphysema, chronic coughing, and other respiratory problems. Only a few will mention heart disease.

Smoking not only is a major risk factor for lung cancer and emphysema but also *doubles* an individual's likelihood of developing heart disease. Smokers with heart disease are up to 70 percent more likely to die of heart disease than are nonsmokers. The heart disease risk increases in relation to the number of cigarettes smoked each day. Individuals who smoke up to 14 cigarettes a day are approximately twice as likely to develop heart disease as those who don't smoke. Those who smoke 15 to 24 cigarettes a day are about four times as likely, and those who smoke more than 25 cigarettes a day are six times as likely to develop heart disease. These statistics, added to the risk statistics for cancer, emphysema, and chronic respiratory diseases, may well shock some people into quitting.

It is not only the smokers who are at risk; secondhand smoke, sometimes called *environmental smoke*, puts nonsmokers at risk, too. Secondhand smoke kills between 37,000 and 40,000 people each year. These statistics from the American Heart Association alone should make every smoker quit and make every household smoke-free! Fortunately, protection from secondhand smoke is now more available, because of new regulations in many states restricting smoking in public places. Unfortunately, children in the home remain unprotected.

I know smoking is bad for my lungs, but why is smoking bad for my heart?

ELEVATED HEART RATE AND BLOOD PRESSURE

There are two especially harmful substances inhaled while smoking. The first is nicotine, the addictive ingredient in cigarettes. When it enters the bloodstream it increases the heart rate, causing the heart to work harder and increasing the need for oxygen in all the cells of the body. Research suggests that nicotine contributes to *arrhythmias* (irregular heartbeats). Smokers' risk of sudden cardiac death is about three times that of nonsmokers'. Nicotine is blamed for elevations in blood pressure while the cigarette is being smoked, which means that a moderate smoker might cause his or her blood vessels to constrict and relax at a rate twenty or so times higher than usual a day. Researchers don't know exactly how this affects the body over time, but they suspect it is damaging. They *do* know that when people already have high blood pressure, smoking makes it more difficult to control.

OXYGEN DEPRIVATION

The second harmful substance is carbon monoxide. Hemoglobin in the blood picks up and delivers oxygen to cells; however, when carbon monoxide is present, it picks up the carbon monoxide *instead*. The cells are unable to utilize it, and they become oxygen-deficient, signaling the heart to work harder to deliver more oxygen. Add this complication to a heart that is already speeded up by nicotine, and you get a worrisome picture. Some researchers believe that carbon monoxide is the element of smoking most likely to cause coronary heart disease. Carbon monoxide is such an enemy of oxygen that if you breathe air high in carbon monoxide for more than a few minutes, you may die. (It is carbon monoxide that kills people who turn on their car engines in a closed garage and sit in the car, breathing that air.)

ATHEROSCLEROSIS

If you have been reading this book sequentially, you've read many times by now about the role of atherosclerosis in heart disease. Atherosclerosis, or the narrowing of arteries due to plaque deposits on artery walls, is considered to be the underlying condition causing coronary heart disease. And smoking, in addition to the other risks it poses for the heart, contributes to atherosclerosis.

Atherosclerotic narrowing of the coronary arteries occurs more often, and more seriously, in smokers than in nonsmokers. And peripheral vascular disease, where the major blood vessels of the arms and legs become narrowed due to atherosclerosis (reducing circulation in the extremities, and sometimes requiring amputation of limbs), is a smokers' disease, occurring infrequently in nonsmokers.

Smoking encourages atherosclerosis in at least two ways. First, it has been shown to lower HDL levels in the blood. HDL, remember, is the "good" cholesterol that helps to carry off fatty wastes to be excreted, as opposed to LDL, the "bad" cholesterol that contributes to plaque formation. Our object should be to raise the HDL level and lower the LDL level. Second, smoking elevates the levels of fibrinogen, a protein, in the blood. High levels of fibrinogen cause the blood to clot more quickly (even when it shouldn't) and can cause clots that adhere to plaque or even obstruct already narrowed blood vessels. A high fibrinogen level is a known risk factor for heart attack and stroke. Smoking causes "sticky blood," or clumping of the platelets, very small particles in the blood that play a key role in blood clotting, and this can lead to clogging of the arteries.

OTHER DAMAGE

Smoking increases the risk of blood vessel spasm, which can be highly damaging or fatal if it occurs in a coronary artery and lasts long enough to cause a heart attack. Smoking can cause hemorrhage (bleeding) in blood vessels. Smoking is known to be a major risk factor for strokes caused by hemorrhage (about 15 percent of strokes). Since smoking is a major cause of lung disease and lung cancer, smokers with heart disease are at greatly increased risk for pulmonary complications, which further damage the heart. Women who smoke and who also take birth control pills multiply their risk of heart disease. And within cigarette smoke itself there are hundreds of compounds, including cyanide, that interfere with the normal life cycle of cells.

Can I lower my risk of heart disease even if I've been smoking for many years?

It's never too late to lower your risk of heart disease. The risk of heart disease rapidly decreases once you stop smoking.

In the first twenty-four hours after quitting, your blood pressure and pulse return to normal, as do the oxygen and carbon monoxide levels in your blood. This alone relieves some of the extra stress you have been imposing on your heart.

Within three months after quitting, you will experience a sharpening of the senses of taste and smell. Your circulation will be improved and your lungs may work at up to 30 percent greater capacity.

After a year, your risk of CHD will be about halfway between a smoker's and a nonsmoker's. Abnormality of blood clotting due to a higher level of fibrinogen (a component of blood that makes blood clotting, possible) and platelets (particles in the blood that by aggregation make the clots possible) related to smoking will disappear, but it takes longer to undo the damage to the arteries. If your smoking has contributed to plaque deposits in the coronary or other arteries, the damage can only be mitigated with time and effort. Combining proper food choices, exercise, and drugs if needed (and even surgery in more extreme cases), you can slowly undo some of this damage.

In three to five years the risk of heart disease, as well as the risk of stroke, will drop to the level of nonsmokers, no matter the number of cigarettes or the years you smoked. Unfortunately, the risk of lung diseases does not subside so quickly, especially if any kind of cancer has started or if some parts of the lungs have already been damaged by emphysema. However, the sooner you stop smoking, the greater your chance of slowing the progress of these diseases, and if you do *not* have these problems already, your risk of lung and oral cancers will continue to decline, reaching the nonsmokers' level in ten to twelve years after quitting.

What makes smoking so addictive? Is it a physical or psychological addiction?

Smoking attracts and holds its devotees by three methods, and it is up to each individual smoker to determine how much each component of addiction affects him or her. Examining this mechanism of addiction not only will help the smoker understand why he or she smokes but will be of assistance once the decision is made to quit.

Nicotine is the *physically addictive* part of cigarette smoke. The potent effects of nicotine go far beyond those of most other legal substances. Nicotine reaches the brain just seconds after it is inhaled and releases chemicals that bring on the sensation of pleasure and a feeling of alertness. Smokers must have a steady supply of nicotine circulating in their blood and going to the brain. Without enough nicotine these sensations begin to diminish, and smokers quickly begin to feel the unpleasant effects of withdrawal, such as headaches, nausea, muscle pain, and insomnia. This is the point at which smokers begin to "crave" a smoke. The degree of nicotine addiction varies from person to person. You can test yours by observing how long you can comfortably go without a cigarette. Those who *must* smoke as soon as they get up in the morning probably have a high level of nicotine dependency.

Nicotine's addictiveness is far beyond that of other substances that may have pleasing psychological or physiological effects. Caffeine, for instance, may become a habit, but many people find it less difficult than nicotine to cut back on, and in most cases it does no harm in moderation.

A cup of coffee or tea in the morning gets us used to caffeine—the physical addiction—and it is also a ritual that we find mentally gratifying—the psychological addiction. Likewise, we become accustomed to associating certain activities, such as drinking coffee or alcohol, finishing a meal, or the proverbial postcoital interlude, with tobacco use. By repetition they become permanently linked as habits. Take note of the activities and environments that cause you to automatically light up, and you will get a glimpse of your psychological addiction.

A *social addiction* to smoking is what motivates many smokers to begin in the first place—the need to fit in with a specific group of people or create a certain kind of image. This is actually a subcategory of psychological addiction, used to distinguish the need to belong from the associative habit described above. Peer pressure leads most smokers to start while still in their teens. Ninety percent of smokers start smoking before they are twenty-one years old.

Is cigar smoking safer than cigarette smoking?

Cigar smoking and smokeless tobacco have been heavily promoted and have increased in use in recent years. Cigar smokers, as well as pipe smokers, differ from cigarette smokers in that they usually do not inhale. It is true that cigar and pipe smoking carries a lower risk of heart disease than cigarette smoking. However, former cigarette smokers who are used to inhaling may inhale when they switch to cigars, even though cigar and pipe smoke is more irritating to the lungs than cigarette smoke. Those cigar smokers who do inhale actually have higher rates of cardiovascular and respiratory diseases than cigarette smokers; and those who don't inhale each puff still passively inhale some of their own secondhand smoke. Whether one inhales or not, the use of cigars and chewing tobacco carries an increased risk of cancers of the mouth and throat, as does inhaling secondhand cigar smoke.

Smokeless tobacco, such as chewing tobacco or snuff, provides a dose of nicotine similar to that of cigarettes—along with the same physical addiction. The routines involved are just as psychologically addicting. The exact risk of heart disease from these substances is not yet known, but because they contain nicotine, they also present a danger to the cardiovascular system. Quitting smokeless tobacco is just as hard as quitting cigarette smoking.

I don't see as many people smoking as I used to. Are people smoking less?

Yes, the number of both men and women smokers has decreased dramatically in the United States since the mid-1960s, when public health messages on the hazards of smoking began to reach the general public. Smoking has declined in the United States by about 35 percent since then. There are currently around 40 million ex-smokers in this country. In some states, like California and Utah, less than 18 percent of adults now smoke. While in the United States smoking is declining, this is not true for other countries where greater affluence is linked to *more* smoking, and where the awareness of the risks of smoking is not as great.

Who smokes more, men or women?

Although more men than women smoke in the United States (26 million men, 23 million women), the rate of decline for male smokers is sharper than that for female smokers: 42 percent of men have quit smoking since 1965 as compared to 32 percent of women. Smoking carries an additional risk of heart attack for women when they also take birth control pills.

What is the best way to quit smoking?

When we interviewed thirty ex-smokers for our book *The Last Puff* (W. W. Norton, 1990), each of them had found his or her own way to quit. You may have to try several different methods to discover what works for you. You or others you know may have already tried to quit, and relapsed. Don't let one or two failed attempts stop you from trying again; many ex-smokers had to try several times to quit. Each failed attempt can be a learning experience, teaching you something you can use on the next try. And if you have decided to quit after experiencing a heart attack or other medical problem, or seeing a friend experience one, your new motivation may be your greatest ally.

What is the first step to quit smoking?

The American Heart Association suggests you set a quit date for yourself, far enough ahead in the future that you have time to prepare yourself. They suggest choosing a significant date to quit—a birthday, job change, or other memorable occasion. On the other hand, many people have successfully quit by just stopping, cold turkey, right now.

The first step is to evaluate your addiction, estimating how much is physical, psychological, and social, as described above. This can help you tailor various smoking interventions to your particular addiction, with its unique physiological, psychological, and social components. To really take a good look at your smoking habit, keep a journal for several weeks, logging each cigarette you smoke. Note the time of day, where you are, who is with you, what you are doing, and your mood. You may learn some surprising things, such as how many cigarettes you really smoke and which situations and moods give you the greatest urge for a cigarette. You may identify some patterns you don't fully understand. This knowledge can help you when you are ready to stop.

What do I do with the information I gather about my smoking habits?

It can be helpful to make a few lists and carry them with you.

- Make a list of situations that most strongly trigger your smoking urge. This will help you recognize them immediately when they occur, or even ahead of time. Work out some advance strategies to respond to this urge, listing some options that might work for you (e.g., leaving the situation, performing some alternative action like gum chewing, taking a walk, eating candy, or saying something prerehearsed to yourself or to others present).
- Decide what you will say when you are offered a cigarette, asked if you've quit yet, or teased. Rehearse these lines often; advocates of the power of positive thinking claim that mental rehearsals are perhaps just as powerful as real-life experiences in the quest to change your behavior.
- Make a list of your motivations to quit so you can reread it whenever you need to.
- Make a list of all your reasons *not* to smoke, including health reasons. This last suggestion is really a form of *aversion treatment*, and you may make the list as detailed and graphic as you wish (even using pictures of lung cancer or emphysema patients and blackened lung tissue if you are so inclined). Aversion treatment works for some people but actually discourages others, so use it only if you feel it will help.

And then, again, you may prefer *not* to make lists. Go with your honest intuition.

What kind of stop-smoking therapies and programs are available?

Quite a few. We'd like to provide statistics about which programs work best, but these are hard to come by and questionable when available. Many programs make inflated claims about their results, and the criteria for "success" are often not defined. Many people quit on their own, with no outside therapies or interventions (we have seen claims that anywhere from 10 percent to 50 percent of ex-smokers quit on their own).

If you have heart disease or other smoking-related problems, your health care professional may be your greatest resource. He or she can refer you to programs and counselors in your area and may know you well enough to have a feeling about what might help most. Your health care professional will also know whether it is advisable for you to try nicotine replacement therapy, which is discussed in more detail later on.

First consider whether you'd like to go into individual counseling with a therapist or would prefer to participate in a group. If you'd like individual counseling, your health care professional or even other ex-smokers may be able to recommend someone. If you prefer group support, you can probably find a local program to help you quit. Some organizations that might offer these include medical clinics and hospitals (some of these will be *for-profit* programs), schools, churches, gyms, state health departments, or community recreation centers.

What about nicotine gums or patches to help people stop smoking?

Although these products are available without a prescription, be sure to discuss their use with your health care professional if you have any symptoms of or risk factors for cardiovascular disease.

Nicotine gum contains about 2 milligrams of nicotine per piece. It is recommended that you chew an average of ten or twelve pieces per day, reducing the number over a period of several months. People with certain heart disorders, ulcers, or throat and mouth problems should not use the gum, so check with your health care professional first. Some people prefer the gum to the nicotine patch because the dose is individually controllable and gives them something to carry around and manipulate. Overuse of the nicotine gum can be a temptation, however, and some people may suffer side effects—burning in the mouth or throat, nausea, and vomiting.

The nicotine patch releases nicotine through the skin and into the bloodstream. It is applied once a day and lasts for either sixteen

SOME POSITIVE REINFORCEMENTS
WHEN YOU DECIDE TO QUIT

- Visualize the recovering function of your heart and lungs (read Chapter 1 if you want specifics about how the heart works). In particular, focus on a lowered heart rate, lowered blood pressure, and full oxygenation of cells, especially the cells of the heart. Think about lower fibrinogen levels in the blood, reducing the "sticky blood" and abnormal clotting conditions. Remember that your risk of arrhythmias is reduced.
- Think of not smoking as a new found freedom from unnecessary, harmful actions. Some protective factors, like exercise or changing your food habits, require action. You need to actively seek out new foods or get out and exercise. But once you have stopped smoking, your job then is to *avoid* something; and you won't even have to buy cigarettes.
- Think of the money you are saving. Consider applying the money you would have spent on cigarettes toward the purchase of something special.
- Consider the positive impact on the health of family and friends.
- Think of yourself as an inspiration to young people not to smoke.
- Enjoy your enhanced appearance. Smoking has been correlated with premature facial wrinkles and dry skin.
- Rediscover the joy of taste and smell. Leslie, a young writer and poet, reminds us that smoking dulls your senses of taste and smell. Writing to a friend about her emotions after she finally quit, following many failed attempts, she describes how during her walks in the park she could now smell the flowers, the spring in the air, and even, at home, something as simple and unpoetic as the scent of freshly washed clothes. Leslie found what everyone who has been a heavy smoker and quit has found: she could smell fragrances and taste things with a new zest.

SOME TECHNIQUES YOU CAN USE TO STAY SMOKE-FREE

- When you are with people who smoke, tell them you have quit and that it would be helpful if they did not smoke around you.
- Watch your alcohol intake; be very moderate—alcohol can weaken your resolve and commitment, and, in many people, calls up associations with smoking.
- If you associate smoking with drinking liquor, switch to wine or beer.
- If you used to smoke in your car, have your car thoroughly cleaned when you quit and designate it as a "no smoking" zone.
- If other people smoke in your family, ask them to smoke outside. Spouses and relatives are usually willing to do so, as they know it affects your health.
- Chew sugarless gum, toothpicks, or straws to keep your hands or mouth busy.
- Follow some of the strategies we talk about in Chapter 9 to reduce stress in your life.
- Go for a walk someplace where smoking is not allowed.
- If you were accustomed to having a cigarette with your morning coffee, try switching to tea or some other hot beverage to help break the association between coffee drinking and smoking.

or twenty-four hours. Those using the twenty-four-hour patch may suffer insomnia or other minor side effects. It is generally used over a period of several weeks to several months, with the amount of nicotine gradually reduced. Again, discuss its use with your health care professional. Some people prefer using the patch to the gum because it is applied only once each day.

People who have a strong physical component to their smoking addiction may find these products useful. They ease withdrawal from the physical addiction to nicotine by delivering it in lower and gradually decreasing doses over time, and they help to break the behavioral links with tobacco use. The nicotine patch and gum release about one fourth as much nicotine into the blood as smoking does. Furthermore, none of those other hundreds of poisons present in cigarette smoke, including cyanide, are present in these products. It is important not to smoke while using them—this can contribute to a heart attack, due to the combined effects of the nicotine inhaled from the smoke and the nicotine in the gum or patch.

Recently some studies have yielded encouraging evidence that some antidepressant medications may be useful in achieving smoking cessation. This new therapy clearly calls for full discussion with your health care professional.

Can you give me some real-life examples I can follow?

When we wrote *The Last Puff*, we interviewed thirty ex-smokers who had successfully quit smoking. Everyone, from business executives to writers, office personnel to truck drivers to lawyers, found the "right" way to succeed. Some had waited so long that a heart attack was the final trigger. But in all cases, the mental and the physical interventions had to work together. Here are two highlights from their stories to help you find your own way to quit.

> For Steve, a college professor, drinking and smoking went together. "My father died of cancer of the esophagus when I was twenty-two [a cancer often caused by heavy drinking of distilled, undiluted liquors and heavy smoking]. I already had a drinking problem and smoked at least a pack of cigarettes a day. My father's death accelerated my drinking and my smoking." Later, Steve tried unsuccessfully to quit smoking many times. Meanwhile he stopped drinking and joined Alcoholic Anonymous, A.A. "The key [to my successful quitting] was to use the A.A. principle: I quit one day at a time. That is what sustained me for the first two years. Then after two years, nonsmoking became a habit, just like smoking used to be."

> Amanda, age thirty-six, a professional dancer and choreographer, had smoked for seventeen years. "Dancers smoke partially to not eat, I think. A lot of dancers have poor eating habits, particularly ballet dancers, and smok-

ing has a lot to do with not wanting to eat." Amanda tried to quit many times. When she moved to the West Coast from New York, she chose to move with her boyfriend into an apartment house in San Francisco where you could not smoke inside the building. She thought that restriction might help, but nothing worked. She had cut down, but not quit. "I was still smoking my six cigarettes a day. After a trip to New York to close my old apartment there, when waiting for a plane at JFK airport, I had one cigarette left in the pack and said, 'That's that,' and that was that. When back in San Francisco, I used techniques I had learned before but never used: I put a sign on my desk, 'Thank you for not smoking' and I would read it and repeat it to myself."

Is it true that the grandson of the founder of a tobacco company quit smoking some years ago?

Yes, Patrick Reynolds, grandson of the founder of R. J. Reynolds Tobacco Company, smoked for ten years. He started because it was against the school rules. He saw his father and many of his relatives, all smokers, die of tobacco-related diseases. Not only did he finally quit (with great effort and after several failed attempts), but he invested his money in the fight against smoking.

9

—

Lifestyle Change: Stress

Stress has been around since the beginning of time. Some of the forms of stress that surround us today are the same as they were centuries ago; others are a product of the evolution of civilization that has brought us such things as traffic congestion. In this chapter you will learn about the various kinds of stress, how their damaging effects are too often overlooked, and how to prevent and relieve stress.

How is stress defined?

The word *stress* itself is a bit confusing in that it is used to describe two aspects of a threatening situation. First, it refers to an outside danger, an incident or situation that alerts you to protect or defend yourself, or to escape. In this sense it is synonymous with "danger," even if the danger is only imagined. The word *stress* also refers to your physical and emotional response to these situations. In a dangerous situation, you might say that you experience stress.

Stress, in its definition as "outside danger," is only partly avoidable, and the truth is you can't always control it. Your body reacts to stimuli that appear to threaten its survival or well-being. The brain perceives danger and reacts by activating physiological mechanisms to defend the body. This is our built-in *fight-or-flight response,* a response that has become one of the foundations of classic teachings in physiology and psychology. The key here is the brain's *perception* of which outside events constitute dangers or stresses.

What happens to the body when it perceives stress?

The body has certain mechanisms to deal with perceived stress that are meant to protect it. Let's say an out-of-control truck is careening toward you and you only have a moment to react. Here are some ways the body will respond to this situation.

The adrenal glands step up their production of stress hormones (adrenaline, noradrenaline, and cortisol) that activate the following responses:

- The metabolism speeds up, i.e., the heart beats faster and pumps more blood, giving you strength, speed, and energy to run or defend yourself.
- Your breathing rate increases, oxygenating the body so that it can work harder and longer.
- Your muscles contract, in preparation for you to spring into action.
- There is an increase in platelet "stickiness" in your blood, causing it to clot more quickly, thus minimizing blood loss in case of injury.
- Your blood pressure rises, probably because your heart is pumping faster and the arteries are constricted, sending more blood to the muscles and brain.
- More blood flows to the arms and legs while less goes to the stomach, giving you energy where you need it most.

This is an example of *acute stress*, where a specific situation causes the body to respond in an appropriate way to protect itself.

So if stress is a natural part of life, what's the problem?

The problem arises when you begin to react as if you were in acute stress too often. Your body can handle these emergency responses in survival situations, but when these responses are activated frequently or for too long a time, they begin to damage the very systems they were designed to protect. When the body is in an ongoing state of reaction to danger, even at a low level, it is said to be in a condition of *chronic stress*.

How does chronic stress affect the body?

That stress, chronic or acute, can lead to a heart attack or another medical crisis has been known for a long time. In chronic stress, stress hormones are present in the body over much greater periods, causing the body's fight-or-flight mechanisms to be activated much of the time. Chronic stress has these effects on the body:

- The heart works harder, beating faster over long periods of time.
- Blood pressure remains higher and, over a long period, can cause damage to the lining of arterial walls, resulting in lesions to which plaque can adhere.
- Since the blood clots more easily, it is easier for clots to form inside the arteries.
- Muscles contract, and potassium and magnesium—nutrients needed for proper artery function—are used up, while sodium and calcium accumulate. This imbalance can result in abnormal artery constriction, including constriction of the coronary arteries, which can cause spasm and perhaps a heart attack.
- Cortisol, a hormone released by the adrenal glands in reaction to stress, causes fat breakdown and circulation of LDL in the bloodstream. In an ongoing stress response, the blood consistently has high hormone and fat levels, potentially contributing to the formation of atherosclerotic plaque.

Stress can have other indirect, insidious effects. It can contribute to increased risk of overeating, heavy smoking, excessive drinking, or apathetic behavior that prevents us from pursuing exercise, a healthy diet, and social interaction.

Can even minor stresses raise blood pressure?

Yes. Just think of all the minor stresses that can be found in a day, from being stuck in traffic to conflicts at work. One example we have all experienced, and one that reminds us how even minor stresses can raise blood pressure, is a visit to a physician's office. In the medical world this is called *white-coat hypertension*. Blood pressure measurements taken in that situation are usually higher than the true average blood pressure, unless the patient has had a chance to rest and relax. This is why at least three measurements are taken in research projects on blood pressure. The patient rests in a quiet environment for a minimum of two minutes after each measurement. Not surprisingly, the last measurement is usually much lower than the first.

Is it true that stressful events can cause heart attacks?

Any cardiologist will tell you that both angina (chest pain) and heart attacks can be triggered by acute stress. Sudden heart attacks happen either because not enough blood and oxygen flow to the heart or because of arrhythmias, erratic or missed heartbeats. If you look at the list of effects of stress on the heart at the beginning of the chapter, you'll see that the heart works harder and arteries constrict, reducing the amount of blood reaching the heart. Ventricular arrhythmias can also be triggered by stress.

It has been suggested that stress may be a trigger for early-morning heart attacks and death from sudden heart attacks and from stroke.

Can I do something about chronic stress?

Remember that stress is just a label. The senses perceive an event or situation, but it is the brain that evaluates the information, interprets it, and labels it as a stress. If the brain labels it stressful, then the body mobilizes its fight-or-flight physiological response. A stress is merely an event or situation that occurs in our environment; we have no control over it. Stress happens. The system of beliefs about *what* is stressful, however, is something over which you do have some control, and it is this belief system you must address in order to alleviate chronic stress.

So what you believe can affect your heart?

If you believe that the traffic jam on the way to work is a stressful event, then your body will come up with the correct stress responses to try to protect you. Only in this case, faster heart rate, higher blood pressure, and constricted muscles and arteries won't do much good; they only make you "stressed." On the other hand, if you see the traffic problem as an event you do not need to defend against, your stress response will not be activated. Thus it makes sense that a person who perceives the government, the IRS, a spouse, or an employer as a continual source of stress in his or her life will live with an ongoing stress response in the body.

What can I do to change my beliefs about what is stressful?

First you must *identify* the things you believe are stressful. A good way to do this is to keep a journal for a few weeks, noting in it everything that causes you stress. Since some of these things may be continual and low-level, it may take some real effort and attention to see them. For example, if you have been feeling stressed by one of your coworkers for the past three years, you may have accepted the way you feel as normal, and may find it difficult to recognize your stress response.

There are other symptoms of stress you will easily recognize once you begin paying attention. You may flush and feel hot; you may develop a headache; you may find yourself breathing rapidly and shallowly; you may experience your heart beating faster; you may feel intense anxiety or worry, or find yourself replaying certain scenarios over and over again. The following list contains physical and emotional responses you may experience when stressed.

PHYSICAL AND EMOTIONAL RESPONSES THAT MAY INDICATE STRESS

Feeling emotionally tense or anxious

Muscle tension

Feeling pressured and rushed

Irritability

Aggressiveness

Worrying all the time

Unable to relax

Unable to plan daily activities

Problems concentrating

Always tired

Constant sadness

Frequent crying

Feeling worthless, insecure

Apathetic about appearance

Sexual apathy

Rapid, shallow breathing

Head, neck, or shoulder pain

Headaches

Jaw tension

Overeating

Not eating enough

Stomach problems

Heavier smoking than usual, or smoking again after quitting

Use of recreational drugs or prescribed medications to relax

Alcohol abuse

Rapid heartbeat

Flushing, feeling hot

If you keep a log for a couple of weeks, using the information and ideas above to help you recognize your stress responses, you should then be able to make a list of the things you believe are stressful in your life.

How can I reduce stress?

Once you have identified the stresses in your life, there are two options available to you to reduce or eliminate them. The first option is to *remove* the stressful elements from your life. If working with a certain colleague is on your list of stress inducers, you could talk to your supervisor about the problem, ask to be transferred, or find a new job. If traffic continually has you on edge, you could look into participating in a car pool or taking public transportation.

The other option is to *change the belief* that working with this particular colleague is stressful, or that traffic congestion causes stress.

There are various ways to work on such attitudinal changes. Affirmation, in which you mentally rehearse the actions and attitudes you wish to adopt, can be helpful. Affirmations are believed by some to "reprogram" negative beliefs already established in your mind. Visualization, in which you imagine the scenario you'd like to become your reality, is a similar method. These methods, while not difficult, require commitment and practice. Many Olympic and professional athletes, as well as many successful businesspeople, pay consultants to teach them and their employees how to incorporate these methods into their work and personal lives. However, it is not necessary to pay a consultant; many books have been written on the subject. Several of these books are listed in the "Suggested Reading" list, and many others are available in most bookstores. You may also wish to seek out a qualified counselor to assist you with these or other attitudinal change therapies, or perhaps join a support group or a medically oriented stress reduction program. (These are often offered through hospitals and clinics.)

What other strategies can I use to reduce stress?

The opposite of stress is relaxation, and any activity that enhances relaxation is a natural stress buster. During relaxation, a number of changes may take place. Often a person's brain waves change from the beta pattern into the alpha pattern, a pattern associated with restful, receptive states of mind. The body requires less oxygen, and the respiratory rate slows. The heart rate slows, blood pressure sometimes declines, and a lower level of stress hormones and cholesterol is present in the blood. Muscle fibers elongate, showing that muscles have relaxed. Anyone with heart disease, or at risk for heart disease, will benefit from these kinds of physiological responses. Two well-known relaxation techniques are yoga and meditation.

YOGA AND DEEP MUSCLE RELAXATION

Yoga is an ancient system of postures, stretches, and breathing exercises designed to bring about health and relaxation. The practice of yoga induces deep muscle relaxation and is very useful for general stress reduction, as it produces mental tranquillity and restores your energy level. Yoga results in real physiological changes: it lowers your pulse rate, decreases your metabolic rate, lowers your blood pressure, and reduces the need for stress hormones that are produced by the adrenal glands.

There are classes, books, and videotapes available to teach yoga to those who wish to learn. There are many styles of yoga, including Kundalini yoga, hatha yoga, and Iyengar yoga, which place varying emphasis on breathing, postures, and types of stretches, so find the type that appeals to you. Other physical relaxation practices emphasizing stretching and breathing, such as T'ai Chi, are valuable as well.

MEDITATION

There are many meditation methods that teach ways to disengage from the constant stream of chatter emanating from the mind. This does not mean you must reject or ignore the mind, only that one can learn to take a step back from it in order to observe its behavior. *Must* you believe everything the mind says? *Must* you continue to defend yourself every time your mind alerts you to stress? Meditation is a tool for investigation. It may surprise you to learn that the presidents and CEOs of some successful high-tech companies take time to meditate every day and also encourage their employees to learn meditation.

When you first begin to practice meditation you may experience stress and frustration when confronted with the mind's ceaseless barrage of mental images, judgments, theories, fantasies, and other ramblings; but with practice, you will be able to block out intruding thoughts and find some peace and quiet. Meditation can help calm you and slow your pulse rate, and is a tool for relaxing even in stressful circumstances. There are many meditation techniques, so look into which one is for you. Prayer, worship, contemplation, and communing with nature also offer the benefits of meditation.

Can exercise reduce stress?

Physical activity is a good way to reduce stress and depression. From walking to swimming, no matter how gentle or how challenging, physical activity is a great healer. Most of us know from experience that exercise makes us feel better psychologically, but scientific support for this belief appeared in *Cardiac Rehabilitation: Clinical Practice*

Guideline, published by the U.S. Department of Health and Human Services in 1995. A panel of experts reviewed various studies and concluded that "exercise training enhances measures of psychological and social functioning . . . including measures of emotional stress." It is known that exercise stimulates production of endorphins, which promote a sense of well-being in the body. Refer to Chapter 10 for more information on appropriate exercise. Find some time for some physical activity, even if only for a few minutes or for a short walk, each and every day.

Is a sense of community important?

It definitely helps to share your feelings. People who don't share their thoughts and feelings, those who hide their distress, who lack social support, often feel isolated or disconnected from others.

Studies have revealed that people who live alone suffer more heart disease than people who don't, and that stress and isolation have a high correlation with death from heart disease. Other studies have found a link between low social support and poorly functioning immune systems.

For an isolated person, finding social support may be stressful at first, just as learning about the workings of the mind may be stressful (see the section on meditation above). After all, people find themselves isolated because relationships can be stressful, so they avoid them. However, now that you have read that isolation is linked to an increased risk of death from heart disease, you may be willing to take some steps to reduce that risk. Therapy groups and emotional support groups are available through churches, schools, community organizations, and medical facilities. If these seem too threatening, consider joining a group that shares some interest of yours, such as books, gardening, philosophy, politics, sports, cooking, or coping with heart disease. Social support and emotional intimacy can facilitate tension release and relaxation, but only you can decide what degree and type of relationships are right for you.

Is it okay to take time for myself?

If some of your stress is triggered by time pressures or the feeling of always being under the gun, then make a special effort to take some time every day to relax. You may need to make yourself a chart to ensure that you include this in your daily routine. Time for yourself is time spent on something that gives you pleasure—it could be cooking, reading, taking a walk, gardening, napping, tinkering, whatever you find enjoyable. Being outdoors exposes you to the healing forces of sun, fresh air, and nature. Or get a massage or other type of bodywork (shiatsu, acupressure, etc.). And don't forget to get enough sleep.

What are stress interventions? Can they be helpful?

An *intervention* is something that "comes between," in this case, something from outside yourself that comes between you and your stress. *Biofeedback* is both a diagnostic and therapeutic tool that can be used to evaluate some of your physiological stress responses, and it can also help you to change them. A technician hooks you up to a biofeedback machine, which uses sensors to monitor your body temperature, muscle tension, brain wave patterns, blood pressure, or heart rate. By learning to recognize which sensations are correlated with body temperature, for example, you can learn to raise and lower the temperature in your extremities by dilating and constricting your blood vessels. You can also learn to tense and relax muscles voluntarily, and to enter different brain wave states at will. Some people learn to control their blood pressure and heart rate to some extent. These skills can be very valuable in inducing relaxation.

Are there any medications that are helpful?

Sometimes medications may be useful in the short term to relieve stress and induce relaxation by lowering heart rate and reducing anxiety and depression. However, the end goal is to learn to relax and cope with stress on your own. Medications should be used only when other relaxation methods, such as yoga, have not been successful and you may still be troubled by sleep disturbances, overwhelming feelings of unhappiness or hopelessness, or difficulty in performing your daily activities. It is then important to consult your physician, who may prescribe specific antidepressant or antianxiety drugs. Beta-blockers are commonly used in people after a heart attack to reduce pulse rate and, to a lesser extent, alleviate anxiety.

Are some people more naturally stressed than others?

There are ways in which some people typically respond to everyday situations, whether stressful or not, that result in physiological reactions that can contribute to heart disease. The strongest association with stress responses is in people who tend to get angry or hostile easily, who are fast-paced, always under time pressures, aggressive, distrustful, or cynical. This type of behavior in a person, familiar to most of us, is called *Type A* behavior.

Books have been written about Type A behavior. People who exhibit this behavior are more likely to have a heart attack than those who are more trusting and calm. There are certain psychological characteristics of a Type A person—such as hostility, cynicism, and anger—that are strongly associated with increased heart attack risk. Those who have a high level of *anger* and *hostility* are at the greatest risk. Anger and hostility may cause the release of hormones such as adrenaline into the bloodstream, which can increase the tendency of blood to clot and raise the blood pressure sufficiently to cause a heart attack. If you feel pressured for time and often hurry or interrupt someone who is speaking to you, you may be a Type A person with an increased risk of heart attack. But you must keep in mind that Type A behavior has been somewhat oversold to the public. It is the anger and hostility part of the Type A personality that is the lethal component. Use stress reduction to relieve this.

Your childhood experiences, your environment over the years, your personal and work life, your successes and failures, the outcome of various events in your life, your general health—and, as always, your genes—all affect the way you respond to stress.

Are you saying that anger, sadness, and other emotions are harmful because they cause stress?

Anger, fear, sadness, and other emotions are a fact of life. Everyone experiences them to some degree or other. Just as physical pain alerts us that something is going on in the body that needs our attention, these painful emotions let us know that something in our psyche needs attention. Sometimes these emotions arise, are acknowledged, and dissipate. At other times, particularly if these emotions are not acknowledged, they arise over and over again until they become a chronic, underlying state. It is when they go unrecognized or are suppressed that emotions become stressful; emotions in themselves are healthy, not harmful.

What about depression — is it the same as stress?

Many of the symptoms of stress are also symptoms of depression, but it is not clear whether depression and stress cause the same physiological responses in the body. It is estimated that between 25 and 30 million Americans suffer from clinical depression (not just moodiness), although many go undiagnosed. The hallmark signs of depression are a loss of interest in life in general and a hopeless, withdrawn, or pessimistic attitude. Depressed people often experience a loss of energy, feel restless, and have trouble concentrating and making decisions. Some do not experience the agitation and rise in blood pressure and heart rate that are part of the stress response; others do. High levels of cortisol are present in many severely depressed patients, contributing to high levels of LDL (the harmful fat in cholesterol) in the blood. If for no other reason than that depression is linked to an elevation in LDL, people with heart disease might want to seek treatment if they think they might be depressed.

It is not uncommon for victims of heart attack or other life-threatening illnesses to experience depression once they are home and recovering. If depressive behavior persists for more than a couple of weeks, it is advisable to seek professional counseling. Medications can help mitigate and interrupt depressive periods, and antidepressants are often prescribed. Patients with heart disease should be sure their doctors are aware of all the medications they are taking, since some depression medications have side effects relevant to heart disease.

Some of the relaxation and belief-modification techniques described above, such as stress avoidance and deep muscle relaxation through yoga, can be very helpful to people experiencing depression.

How do I get started with stress management?

STEP 1: IDENTIFY THE STRESSORS IN YOUR LIFE AND THE EMOTIONS THEY BRING OUT

These stresses may be deadlines, overwork, financial pressures, family or marital difficulties, lack of support in daily activities, relationships with coworkers, child-rearing, housework, etc. Once you identify the major issues in your daily life, you'll be on the path to reducing the toll they take on you and your health. Then determine what emotions they trigger. Does the daily traffic jam make you tense or angry? Does being late make you feel inadequate? Does a disagreement with other people in your family make you feel hostile or unloved?

Here is the story of Maggie and how she successfully managed to decrease stresses in her complex life.

Maggie is in her late fifties and has high blood pressure and a high blood cholesterol level; she has grown children in college and a retired husband at home. She is the marketing vice president of a major retail company. She took her first step in stress relief by identifying the biggest stressors in her life to be her job, followed by finances—she has two kids in college—and the lack of support she gets from her husband, who seems indifferent to her problems. She always feels under pressure, overburdened, and too short on time. She is usually tense, irritated, sometimes hostile, and by the end of the day she is sad, disappointed, feeling inadequate, and depressed.

After reading this book, she tries to follow some of the suggestions on stress management and relaxation.

STEP 2: BREAK THE CHANGEABLE STRESSORS INTO SMALLER MANAGEABLE PIECES

This is the time to determine which stresses can be changed and which are unchangeable. Make a list of the stresses in your life over which you have some control. These are the stresses you can eliminate or modify, such as joining a car pool rather than experiencing the stress of traffic congestion on your way to work. (We will talk later about those things that can't be changed.) Begin with one or two things over which you know you have control. Break up big things into smaller parts that will be easier to tackle.

Maggie begins to keep a record of the activities surrounding her job and her feelings associated with it for a few typical days. She learns that she always feels tired in the morning, and usually gets up with great difficulty when the alarm clock goes off. Often she oversleeps. This sets off a rush to get ready, triggering negative thoughts about the entire day. She makes a note of this on her stressors list.

The traffic on the way to work always seems too slow to her and she is angry with the other drivers on the freeway. By the time she gets to work, she feels harried and rushed. She keeps her own calendar but has never considered adjusting her schedule to manage her time. She often skips lunch or a lunchtime break, becoming fatigued and irritable in the afternoon. Constant interruptions often lead to work not getting done. By the time she returns home, she is tired, but the sum of all her tensions frequently leads to insomnia lasting several hours every night. The result is that Maggie wakes up not rested enough and feeling exhausted and depressed, and then starts the cycle all over again.

She decides that one of the first and easiest things to do would be to set up a plan for reducing the tension and anger she experiences in traffic each day. She realizes that she has complete control over her own environment in the car but cannot do anything about other people's actions in traffic. She decides to play tapes of mystery novels—one of her mental escapes—in her car. They keep her mind occupied to the point where soon she does not mind the traffic jams and is so focused on the story that she almost hopes for more time to listen!

Maggie learned that by lessening her anger in traffic, she can reduce her feelings of stress. She begins to see things in a different light. The plantings along the road remind her of her garden at home—she starts using the time to plan her seasonal planting. Then she discovers she can use the time in the car to evaluate her day at work, or to review presentations and reports for which she is responsible.

STEP 3: REVIEW YOUR PROGRESS DAILY AND REVISE YOUR PLAN AS NEEDED

For at least the first few weeks, keep a daily record of your responses to your new plan. It takes time for a new behavior to become habit and often a few months before it really becomes routine. Ask yourself, "How stressed did I feel today after implementing my plan?" Give yourself a rating on a scale of 1 to 5, with 1 being not stressed at all. Your goal will be to have a low score most of the time.

After you determine how you have been doing, be flexible and be willing to revise your goals or add new ones. Of great importance is being open to reidentifying the problems—you may see them differently this time. It is often useful, as well as motivating, to identify unexpected benefits of your plan.

> *Maggie's evaluation for the first month was very positive and fruitful. And she noted other unexpected benefits: she arrived at work more refreshed and alert with more energy, which enabled her to work more efficiently during the day and to interact with coworkers more positively and successfully. She found that some tasks took less time as her mind was more relaxed and she had not wasted energy worrying about the traffic situation, which she could not change anyway.*

On the other hand, after you have reviewed your initial attempts at stress management, you may find that you have set unrealistically high standards for yourself. This is the time to be open to returning to the first step and to be flexible about reassessing the stressors in your life. Some people may have to go through this process a few times before they find the proper routine. People who learn how to manage stress generally have a much easier time making and sticking to other changes, such as changing their diet, getting exercise, or quitting smoking, than those who ignore the insidious nature of stress. People who learn how to manage stress tend to find their lives more enjoyable. They generally feel better and are often able to accomplish more.

> *Maggie now decided to tackle her financial stress. With two children in college and a husband on a fixed income, and feeling there was no possibility of advancement in her job, Maggie saw no way to increase her income. Close to retirement herself, she was unwilling to change her career. She was also unwilling to ask her children to drop out of school, even for a year. What could she do?*
>
> *Recognizing that she had run out of ideas, Maggie decided to address her belief that she was in financial "danger." Although skeptical, she decided to give affirmation and visualization a try. She wrote this message on an index card, which she read to herself every morning and evening and whenever else she remembered to: "I am safe and secure. Whatever happens is for my*

benefit. I have done my best for my family and myself, and I welcome whatever changes come into my life." *At the same time, she pictured herself and her husband strolling the streets of London, a city she had always wanted to visit but felt was too expensive.*

Did Maggie inherit a million dollars and visit Buckingham Palace? We don't know, but we do know that within several months she no longer considered herself financially deprived. She felt open to new adventure.

STEP 4: THE SELF-REWARD STRATEGY

An optional step in this process, which for some people is highly effective, is to use a self-reward. This is a very personal strategy. Some individuals find the satisfaction that comes with successfully fulfilling their own goals so rewarding that nothing more is necessary. Others find the simple measure of promising themselves something special adequately motivating.

The kind of self-reward someone chooses is highly personal. Self-rewards can be anything from the promise of seeing a new movie to an elaborately planned vacation. Think seriously about the potential of including self-reward in your stress management plan.

10

Lifestyle Change: Exercise

The human body was created to be physically active: in earlier centuries we had no choice but to do physical work, to walk much more than we do today, to gather and prepare our own food. In industrialized countries the need for physical activity has been reduced to a minimum, and it is therefore imperative that we make exercise a regular routine in our lives. In this chapter you will read about the various types of exercise and how to approach them if you have heart disease. You will see how crucial a component of good health exercise is.

Why is exercise so important?

The heart, like our other muscles, needs to be kept in good condition. The regular pumping that keeps us alive—for most people this means blood pumping in and out of the heart about 60 to 80 times every minute—is not enough to keep the muscle tuned and the coronary arteries clean. Tuning up the heart is simple: you need to increase its number of beats or pumping cycles at least a few times a week for a minimum of twenty to thirty minutes each time. If you are not well enough to engage in strenuous activity, even some easy physical activity like walking for a reasonable length of time will help the tune-up process.

Using muscles for physical tasks was a daily necessity in primitive societies. Humans were able to endure long bouts of exercise and exposure to heat and cold while seeking and gathering plants, hunting, and fishing. Skeletal analyses of primitive human remains indicate that the early human was an extraordinarily active creature whose bones were as strong as those of a modern conditioned athlete. From this we can infer that the early human's cardiovascular system was in pretty good shape as well.

The sedentary lifestyle typical of contemporary society is a major risk factor for heart disease. Inactivity contributes to obesity, diabetes, and high blood pressure, which we already know are correlated with heart disease and lead to fatigue, stress, and often depression.

What will I gain by exercising?

- Studies have shown that regular aerobic exercise lowers triglycerides, increases HDL (the good cholesterol), and sometimes reduces LDL (the bad cholesterol).
- Over time, exercise can increase the size of the coronary arteries and the capillaries that supply blood and oxygen to the heart. Some evidence exists that exercise may even promote the formation of extra blood vessels to help compensate for those that are blocked.
- Exercise helps control blood pressure. If your blood pressure is normal, physical activity will help it stay that way. If it is elevated, exercise can help lower it.
- Exercise helps control blood sugar and prevent non-insulin-dependent diabetes.
- Exercise helps prevent blood clotting in arteries and veins.
- Exercise improves your overall quality of life. As your heart works more efficiently, it does so with less effort. You'll find you have more energy.
- Exercise helps with weight loss and weight control. A physically active person burns more calories while exercising and *even when resting*.
- Exercise strengthens bones and muscles.
- Exercise helps you respond to stress.
- Exercise reduces depression.

• Exercise improves your body's appearance. You look fit and strong, which can do wonders for your self-image.

Exercise may be healthy, but how will it slow down or reverse my heart disease?

Studies have shown that regular exercise lowers the risk of death from a second heart attack; there are about half as many heart attacks among people who exercise, as among those who don't. Studies also show that heart disease risk factors such as blood cholesterol, triglycerides, lipids, high blood pressure, and obesity are lowered in people who get regular aerobic exercise. Angina attacks decrease in heart disease patients who follow an exercise program. Exercise has also been shown to improve glucose tolerance and retard the development of non-insulin-dependent diabetes.

Exercise is also good for the heart muscle itself. When you do regular aerobic exercise, the heart beats faster, indicating that it is working harder—that is, you are exercising the heart muscle. This causes an increase in the size of the muscle, and the amount of blood flowing to it. As the muscle strengthens, it can pump more forcefully, causing even more blood and oxygen to circulate with every stroke. A strong heart, during rest periods, beats fewer times per minute than a weaker heart, allowing more time in each interval for oxygen and nutrients to be absorbed by the heart and other organs and tissue.

I've tried exercise programs before and failed. How can I keep myself from giving up?

This time it's different, because now you know that your health and your life are at stake, a tremendous motivation for all heart disease patients. You can use this motivation to make exercise a *habit* in your life, an automatic behavior that is accomplished almost without conscious intervention.

It takes time for a new behavior to become a habit. Behavioral scientists have found that it takes twenty-one days to establish a pattern and about fourteen weeks (or a hundred days) of repeating the behavior to make it an automatic routine. The first month is usually the most difficult for people who were not physically active before

TIPS TO HELP YOU ESTABLISH
YOUR EXERCISE HABIT

- **Start slowly.** Too much, too soon, too fast can lead to medical problems, fatigue, and other negative consequences, as well as increase chances of injury.
- **Choose activities that are pleasurable.** If you get bored or the activity is inconvenient, you may not exercise regularly. Remember, there are many exercise options, and it's okay to experiment.
- **Choose a variety of activities.** Vary your routine—walk one day, swim another day.
- **Set goals** that work for you—gradually incorporate them into your daily activity.
- **Keep an exercise diary** at first to see if you have met your goals.
- **Schedule exercise times.** Consider them a commitment, like a business or social appointment. Make these times convenient.
- **Get some support.** Enlisting a friend or companion is often helpful, particularly when—as happens to everyone—motivation sags or interest lags.
- **Join a walking club.** It's a good way to meet people who share your health-oriented goals.
- **Get expert help.** Many gyms, community recreation departments, community colleges, senior centers, and the YMCA have exercise counselors.
- **Be sure you have comfortable gear.** Wear clothes that fit comfortably and are appropriate for the weather and activity. Wear good-quality, comfortable shoes.
- **Alternate** aerobic exercise with strengthening activities to protect your feet and legs and to add variety. Remember that *variety is the spice of life;* and if your physical activities are interesting, you are more likely to do them regularly.
- **Go out and do it!**

their diagnosis. This is where your newfound motivation will help. Give yourself small daily goals to achieve, such as doing your errands on foot instead of by car. Your body might complain at first, but you will enjoy the prospect of extra years of health. Usually those who get beyond the hundred-day threshold period stand a good chance of making exercise an activity they *want* to do rather than one they *must* do.

What is the best kind of exercise for me?

There are three types of exercise: aerobic, resistance, and stretching. The word aerobic comes from the Greek word for air, and it refers to any regular, rhythmic exercise using the legs or arms that requires an increased breathing rate over a period of time. Aerobic exercise is what is needed to strengthen the cardiovascular system. Some aerobic activities are

- swimming
- fast walking
- jogging
- bicycle riding

Resistance exercise, important for building muscle and keeping it strong, draws largely on energy stored in muscles and does not require nearly as much oxygen. Resistance exercise involves activities in which the muscles meet resistance, such as in weight training or muscle conditioning. Lifting *light* weights with many repetitions versus using heavy weights with fewer repetitions will strengthen muscles at a steadier rate with less risk of injury. You can begin doing resistance exercises at home by lifting commonplace objects such as soup cans.

Resistance exercise should be part of a healthy lifestyle to help keep muscles and bones strong and prevent hip and other bone fractures. When done properly, this type of exercise should pose little risk to your heart. However, avoid lifting heavy weights as this may lead to potentially dangerous increases in blood pressure. You must be the judge of what is excessive weight, as it is linked to your previous weight training.

Stretching keeps the muscles flexible. Stretching before engaging in any aerobic or resistance exercise is important, as it helps prevent injuries. Stretching is also a good way to relax. Yoga is an ancient Asian art that involves a lot of stretching. A good class in yoga or a related type of exercise, such as T'ai Chi, can help keep your muscles fit and relax you as well. Once you've learned these stretches, you can do some every day at home.

The greatest benefit to the heart comes from aerobic activity. It uses large muscles to get the heart pumping and the lungs filling with oxygen. Resistance exercise and stretching keep your muscles strong and flexible so you can continue your aerobic activity.

Is there any risk in exercising with heart disease?

Exercise has lots of benefits, but there are some risks. How much or how little you should do depends on your diagnosis. If you have survived a heart attack or have had heart surgery, you should first talk to your health professional about supervised exercise in an organized cardiac rehabilitation program. This chapter will build on what you learn in cardiac rehabilitation and provide you with tools to maintain a safe and healthy exercise program. Whatever the severity of your heart disease, you should discuss exercise with your physician or health professional before beginning any program.

In addition, your physician may have prescribed medication such as beta-blockers (a type of blood pressure medication discussed in Chapter 5) that limits the body's ability to increase the heart rate. (Not all drugs affect your ability to exercise or to increase your heart rate.) When your physician prescribes *any* medication, discuss how exercise might affect it.

If exercise is supposed to be so good for you, why do some young athletes die suddenly of heart attacks?

This is almost always because the young person has a different kind of heart disease, called *cardiomyopathy*. This problem is not due to atherosclerosis and most often has no known underlying cause. It is another cause of congestive heart failure and occurs most often in adults, preceded by many months of shortness of breath. Fortunately deaths from cardiomyopathy are relatively rare (about one in fifty of all cases of heart disease).

What can I do to make my exercise program as safe as possible?

First and foremost, discuss exercise with your physician. This is a *must* if you have heart disease or known risk factors for heart disease. Check with your physician and get clearance—ask what you should or should not be doing. After reading this chapter, you'll know what questions to ask. *It's essential that you communicate to your physician that you want to become physically active.*

What if I have arthritis?

If you have arthritis, learn how to do gentle stretching and flexibility exercises or underwater aerobics, which often allows exercise without pain.

How do I design a safe exercise program?

There are four parts to a safe exercise program:

- warming up
- working out
- avoiding overexertion
- cooling down

Why is warming up so important?

Prior to any stretching activity, it is preferable to warm up. The purpose of the warm-up is to raise the core body temperature and lubricate the joints. "Cold" muscles are more susceptible to injury, even in a very well-conditioned individual. Furthermore, when muscles are stretched while warm, greater increases in flexibility can be achieved and maintained than if stretching is done without a prior warm-up. The warm-up need last only five minutes. It can consist of walking, riding a stationary bicycle, working out on a rowing machine, or using any other type of exercise equipment involving rhythmic movements of the large muscle groups of the body. If more convenient, a warm shower or bath may substitute as a warm-up.

A SIMPLE, SAFE STRETCHING PROGRAM (no equipment needed)

Front Shoulder/Chest

"Shoulder roll and reach for the sky"

To increase the benefits of this stretch, shoulder rolls can be performed first, five forward and five reverse:

Raise shoulder to ears; bring shoulders back (retract shoulder blades); lower shoulders; bring shoulders forward.

Now "reach for the sky" with both arms about three or four times.

Upper Back/Neck

Interlace fingers, turn palms from body, and push hands outward at chest level until arms are fully extended. Hold position for 15 to 30 seconds. Repeat two or three times.

Lower Back (lumbar spine)

Kneel on your hands and knees. Raise your back in an arching curve (like a cat when it stretches) and hold this position for 5 seconds.

Now dip your back in the opposite direction (like the dip between the humps on a camel's back) and hold this position for 5 seconds.

Repeat the "cat and camel" positions one or two more times.

Hip Flexors

Find a firm, supportive surface on which to lie on your back, such as a carpeted floor or exercise mat.

From this position, pull your right knee to your chest, keeping fingers interlaced behind your right leg. Slowly straighten your left leg along the mat or floor as much as possible. Hold this position for 15 to 30 seconds. Repeat with the left leg pulled to the chest while straightening out the right leg along the floor or mat. Do once for each leg.

Note: If you have back problems, be cautious. This routine may need to be modified. Check with your instructor or a health professional.

Calves

Standing about eighteen inches from a wall, feet about hip-width apart, place your hands on the wall. Your hands should be at shoulder level, but spaced wider than the shoulders. Bring your right foot back as much as possible while keeping the right heel down and toes pointing ahead. The left knee should automatically bend to accommodate this position. If more of a stretch is needed, slowly lean into the wall, bending the elbows, until a stretch is felt in the calf area. Hold position for 15 to 30 seconds. Repeat for the left leg. Do once for each leg.

Hamstrings (hamstring group, back of thigh)

Note: There are many ways to stretch the hamstrings, but most positions require a significant degree of flexibility. The following stretch accommodates the least flexible individual and allows for any gains made in flexibility.

Sit on a bench (an exercise bench is ideal), toward one end, so that your legs are straddling the bench. Swing your right leg onto the bench so that it is extended on the bench (your left foot remains on the floor). Your right leg should be straight, but if this is not possible, you can bend your knee, with the goal being to eventually straighten your leg along the bench. Likewise, in cases of extreme inflexibility, you may have to lean back while holding onto the sides of the bench for support. This is fine.

Conversely, if an increased stretch is desired, slowly lean into your leg without rounding your back, until you feel a stretch in the back of your thigh. Hold the position for 15 to 30 seconds.

Repeat this for your left leg. Do once for each leg.

An even simpler beginning hamstring stretch (called "Good Morning") involves bending forward at the waist while standing with your hands on your hips. Bend at the waist with your back straight until you feel a pull in the back of your thigh (in the hamstring muscles). Bend and straighten ten to twenty times. This exercise also strengthens the muscles of the lower back.

How do I choose an aerobic exercise program?

If you have heart disease, are at high risk for heart disease, or have not been exercising, it is important to start slowly and build up your exercise program gradually. Gentle stretches and short walks are a good way to begin. As you begin to feel stronger, you can lengthen your walks and incorporate some uphill segments. If you decide to take the stairs instead of the elevator, take them slowly at first, resting whenever you need to catch your breath.

In choosing a form of exercise, keep in mind that in order to be aerobic it must be regular and rhythmic, require an accelerated breathing rate over the duration of the exercise, and use the large muscles of the arms and/or legs. It is an advantage to practice more than one kind of regular exercise, since different muscle groups are toned and stretched by different exercises.

There are hundreds of exercise options, and the key to picking the "best" one for you is to pick one—or several—that you really enjoy doing. This may require some experimentation, particularly if you did not exercise regularly before your heart disease diagnosis. You have a far better chance of succeeding with your exercise program if you're enjoying yourself.

How often should I exercise?

Your goal should be to exercise three to five times a week, for twenty to thirty minutes at a stretch. However, if time allows, exercising daily is even better. But don't be concerned if you do not make the

---

THINGS TO CONSIDER IN DECIDING WHAT KIND OF EXERCISE IS RIGHT FOR YOU

- **Social interaction**
  Do you prefer to exercise *alone* (for instance, swimming, jogging), *in competition with one or two others* (tennis, racquetball), *on a team* (softball, basketball), *or in a class situation* (such as a low-impact aerobic exercise class)? Many communities now offer exercise classes for people with heart problems—check your local recreation programs and health services.

- **Environment**
  Do you want to be indoors or outdoors? In a gym, on a court, track, or playing field, or out in nature?

- **Financial**
  How much money are you prepared to spend? Consider the costs of gym membership, ski equipment, good athletic shoes, etc. For walking, all you need to buy is a pair of supportive walking shoes—a minimal expense for better health!

---

full thirty minutes at first—you will, with practice and time. Don't make exercise an all-or-nothing situation. Even five minutes a few times a day is better than no exercise at all. It has been shown that short periods of exercise, even five minutes, are still beneficial, especially when they add up to at least twenty minutes per day. After a few weeks you will likely notice that moving around is easier. Then you will need to work a little harder to elevate your heart rate. This is a good sign, for it means that your heart is becoming stronger.

How hard should I exercise?

You need to get your heart beating fast enough to be of benefit but not so fast as to be potentially harmful. Your most beneficial heartbeat rate is called your *target heart rate*. It is a straightforward matter for you to determine your target heart rate and to monitor your actual heart rate during exercise. This is an essential element of your exercise program, because exceeding your target heart rate can be dangerous, and failing to achieve it can limit the benefit of the exercise.

How do I determine my target heart rate?

To calculate your target heart rate, subtract your age from 220, which gives you the number of beats per minute you would achieve during *maximal, all-out effort* while exercising. This is referred to as your *maximum heart rate*. The *optimal heart rate* for maximum benefit is *between 70 percent and 80 percent* of your maximum heart rate. This means that a sixty-five-year-old woman or man with a maximum heart rate of 155 (220 - 65 = 155) has *a target heart rate of between 109 and 124 beats per minute* (70 to 80 percent of 155). You can use the table below to quickly find your approximate target heart rate, but the most accurate way is to use the formula given above.

To find out if you are in your target range, take your pulse immediately after you stop moving. Don't delay, as your pulse rate typically drops rapidly. Learn how to find your own pulse: place two fingers—don't use your thumb, because it has a pulse of its own—on the inside of your wrist. Count the beats for 10 seconds (practice taking your pulse until it becomes easy). Then multiply by 6 to get heartbeats per minute. If the sixty-five-year-old person in the example

Table 10–1. Approximate Target Heart Rates

Age	Target Heart Rate	
	70% max.	80% max.
20–24	138.6	158.4
25–29	135.1	154.4
30–34	131.6	150.4
35–39	128.1	146.4
40–44	124.6	142.4
45–49	121.1	138.4
50–54	117.6	134.4
55–59	114.1	130.4
60–64	110.6	126.4
65–69	107.1	122.4
70–74	103.6	118.4

above had a 10-second pulse of 20 beats (20 times 6 equals 120 beats per minute), it would fall within the target heart rate range of 109–124. (Inexpensive watchlike devices that you wear on your wrist are available to electronically measure your heart rate if you find that helpful.)

Another way to do this is to divide your target heart rate by 6, which gives you a 10-second value. In the above example the target heart rate would be between 18 and 21 (109–124 beats per minute divided by 6 yields a range of 18–21 beats per 10 seconds). Then when you take your pulse, it will be immediately obvious whether your pulse falls into the target heart rate range. If it is lower than your target rate, you will know that next time you need to either increase the amount of effort used or the length of time spent exercising. If your pulse is higher than your target rate, then next time slow down until it falls into the proper range. In the beginning especially, take your pulse often to get a sense of how your body is responding. As you get into better shape and continue exercising, however, you may find that you can estimate your heart rate based on the way your body feels.

What if something goes wrong? How will I know if I need medical help?

You should always be free of pain and able to move and talk comfortably and to breathe regularly and rhythmically. If you can carry on a normal conversation, then it's likely that your heart rate is not too high.

The maxim "No pain, no gain" is a myth; and it can be a dangerous myth for someone with heart disease. If you sense any pain, you know you're exercising improperly or something is going wrong. Whatever physical activity you do should take some effort, but real pain is a sign that your muscles and your heart are working too hard or in the wrong way. Stop immediately whenever you feel pain, and don't resume that activity until you can do so without pain.

Why do I need to cool down after exercising?

At the end of any physical workout that raises your heart rate, you should slow down gradually rather than coming to a sudden stop.

Stop exercising immediately and talk with your physician if you experience any of the following:

- chest pain or any chest discomfort
- shortness of breath with only moderate physical activity
- any pain or discomfort in your arm, neck, or jaw
- headache or dizziness
- nausea

This gives your heart a chance to decrease its rate gradually and helps prevent a sharp drop in blood pressure, which can happen if you stop abruptly. It also helps to reduce muscle stiffness.

How do I cool down?

In modern gyms, many treadmills or other aerobic exercise machines are programmed to slow down for at least one or two minutes before stopping. You should also slow from jogging or fast walking to a normal pace for at least five minutes. Follow your workout with a few minutes of gentle stretching using the exercises we've designed (see box on pages 108–10). If you plan an easy walk, a slow swim, or other nonstrenuous physical activity, warming up and cooling down are not as important.

Can you give me some ideas for putting extra activity into my day?

There is much more you can do to increase your physical activity beyond formal exercise routines. You are surrounded by gadgets—from elevators to power lawn mowers to TV remote controls—designed to reduce physical labor. Here are ideas to help you add more physical activity to your days. Not only will you help your heart but you will control your weight as well.

- Slightly exaggerate your movements, by slowly stretching, when you garden or clean house.

- Go back to using hand-powered household tools and appliances—a whisk, a manual rotary beater, a carpet sweeper—instead of electrical ones, unless you have arthritis.
- Use a push mower instead of a power or ride-on mower to cut your lawn.
- Hide the television remote control so that you must get up to change channels.
- Use stairs, rather than elevators and escalators, whenever possible.
- Park at the far end of the parking lot.
- Walk your dog.
- Take short, periodic walk breaks at work, even if it is just around the building or the floor you are on.

11

—

Lifestyle Change: Diet

Your choice of foods is one of the most powerful tools you have at your disposal to help in your recovery from heart disease and in preventing a future heart attack. A few simple guidelines will make choosing foods that are good for you easy. Fortunately it's getting easier and easier to find healthy foods in many restaurants, cafeterias, and supermarkets. More farmers' markets have a wide array of fresh, convenient, and appealing vegetables and fruits that make the preparation of the ultimate, healthful meal a joy rather than a chore.

Other heart-healthy lifestyle changes may mean learning new skills. You may need to learn to exercise if you have always been sedentary, and you may have to learn to deal with stress, but you already know what a delight eating can be. What you may need to learn is how to add some new food choices to your diet, and how to make these choices enjoyable. It may seem a lot of trouble to experiment with new foods at this point in your life. But once you've changed your eating habits, you will be making your heart healthier and your whole body will feel better.

Will the foods I choose for my heart help prevent other diseases, too?

Recent research shows that the kinds of foods you should eat for heart health are the very foods that may prevent many cancers, the number two killer in Western countries.

Will I have to be on a diet for the rest of my life?

For some of us, the term *diet* is synonymous with restriction and deprivation; to others it is synonymous with hospitals, illness, boring, bland dishes, and an inquisitive scientist looking over everything you eat. So forget "dieting"! The term *diet,* in its true sense, is "a way to eat," not a weight loss regimen.

Choose some great foods that taste good. Forget counting calories and measures of fat! Rather, learn to enjoy the right foods in a new way. Maybe, for a few days or weeks, you'll have to make a conscious effort to choose healthy foods and eliminate others, but soon you'll feel free and happy, and your new "diet" will not look like a diet anymore. You'll wonder how you could possibly have eaten any other way!

Is there a simple formula for a heart-healthy diet?

Yes, there are three key steps:

- Increase your consumption of plant foods like vegetables, whole grains, beans and lentils, seeds and nuts, fresh and dried fruits.
- Eat these foods in forms as unrefined as possible.
- Decrease your consumption of animal products, especially high-fat animal products.

It is good to keep things simple, and a good way to start is to make yourself two lists: one of foods to eliminate from or reduce in your diet and one of foods to add or consume in larger amounts. The table below will help you to make the proper choices.

Is it true that fat is bad for me?

Fat is one of the most misunderstood components of foods. It is wrong to say that fat is good or neutral or bad, because fat is not a

Table 11-1. Heart Disease Risk Reduction Foods

Increase or add	Decrease or eliminate
• Whole grain products such as whole grain breads and other whole grain baked products, whole grain pastas and cereals, brown rice, barley, oats, and other whole grains • Beans and bean products, lentils, peas, and their products • Soybean products: tofu, tempeh, soy milk, and miso • Fresh and dried fruits of all kinds • Vegetables of all kinds, raw and cooked, and vegetable juices • Foods rich in unsaturated fats such as all tree nuts, nut butters, and nut oils; olives and olive oil; avocados; sesame, sesame oil, and tahini; sunflower seeds and sunflower oil; peanuts and peanut butter when free of partially hydrogenated fats • Foods rich in omega-3 fatty acids such as flaxseed, walnuts, and all fishes	• Refined flour products, such as white breads and baked products, white pasta • Foods high in saturated fat like meat, poultry, especially sausages and luncheon meats unless a low-fat content is stated on the label; high-fat milk products; and coconut • Foods with partially hydrogenated oils, found in many baked products, some margarines, most processed and convenience foods, and in fast foods • Animal foods high in cholesterol, present mostly in the fat of all meats and poultry and in egg yolks • Foods fried in unknown fats such as many commercial French fries and fried chips, unless unsaturated fat is listed on the label

single chemical entity but rather a mixture of related compounds that can have quite different effects on your health. What is true is that some fats can raise blood cholesterol while others do not raise it. This is especially crucial for someone with heart disease. There is a difference between saturated and unsaturated fats. Every food contains a mixture of saturated and unsaturated fat, but their relative amount varies greatly: some foods are high in saturated fats, others are high in unsaturated fats.

What's the difference between saturated and unsaturated fats?

Most saturated fats raise blood cholesterol or keep it high if it is elevated, while natural unsaturated fats do not raise blood cholesterol and, when replacing saturated fat in the diet, lower it. This has been proven in hundreds of clinical studies. If you are a chocolate lover there is good news for you: the natural saturated fat in chocolate, called stearic acid, does not raise blood cholesterol.

On the other side, one type of unsaturated fat does not lower blood cholesterol: the partially hydrogenated type you find in many processed foods. Here the chemical structure of the fat has been twisted in such a way that it not only does not lower blood cholesterol but sometimes even raises the bad cholesterol and lowers the good cholesterol.

I know I must cut down on saturated fats, but what about cholesterol in foods?

Cholesterol has many roles in human health. For example, some hormones and bile acids are synthesized from cholesterol, and cholesterol is part of the cell wall. But your body makes all the cholesterol you need, so you do not need to get more from foods. Up to a point, cholesterol from foods does not alter your blood cholesterol, but above a certain level, in most people, it *raises* blood cholesterol. A few people can eat more, with no damage, but if you have heart disease, you must be extra careful.

Cholesterol is found only in animal foods, and most often it is dissolved in the fat part of the food. If you decrease the amount of animal fat you eat, you decrease your cholesterol intake as well. As you know, two of the richest sources of cholesterol in foods are egg yolks (egg whites have no cholesterol) and liver (cholesterol is synthesized in the liver). You can eat low-fat animal foods in moderation, such as nonfat or low-fat yogurt, which contain almost no cholesterol. Cholesterol in food is even worse for your health when eaten in combination with high saturated fats. Never eat whole eggs with food high in saturated fat like butter or breakfast meats.

Try not to consume more than 200 milligrams of cholesterol per day—about one small egg yolk or 6 or 7 ounces of cooked beef, chicken, or pork. If you eat eggs, eat the white only (it is also a good protein source) and limit egg yolks to no more than two a week. Try to avoid liver altogether.

Are there foods that can lower cholesterol?

Yes. Plants contain substances related to cholesterol called sterols, which, instead of raising blood cholesterol, actually lower it. Before modern cholesterol-lowering drugs, there were medications available that used plant sterols to lower blood cholesterol. They work by decreasing the absorption from the intestine of the cholesterol present in animal foods.

Foods high in plant sterols are

- tree nuts and their products, such as almonds, Brazil nuts, cashews, hazelnuts, macadamias, pecans, pine nuts, pistachios, and walnuts
- seeds and their products, such as sesame, sunflower, and pumpkin seeds; peas, peanuts, soybeans, kidney beans, and broad beans
- olives and extra virgin unfiltered olive oil
- wheat germ and whole wheat products, the germs of other grains, and rice bran

A few margarines (Benecol, Take Control) are now available that are enriched with a modified form of plant sterols.

Are there other heart benefits from plant foods?

The proteins in plants are much higher than animal proteins in an important amino acid—one of the building blocks of proteins—called *arginine*. Arginine relaxes the arteries and may help to lower cholesterol. Nuts, beans, whole grains, and soy products are high in arginine.

All natural plant foods are high in potassium and magnesium and low in sodium, which help in blood pressure control. Some foods like kale, collard greens, and broccoli are high in calcium, which is needed for proper heart function. This means you don't have to count just on yogurt and other milk products for your calcium.

Should I make foods like whole grains, beans, nuts, fruits, and vegetables the foundation of my meal?

Yes. Some very good studies have shown that when people move from countries where the diet is based on these kinds of foods to countries where the diet is based on meat and other animal products, and where plant foods play only a supporting role, the incidence of heart disease—and some other chronic diseases like colon cancer—increase. A classical example is that of Japanese people moving from Japan to Hawaii with a moderate increase in heart disease, and then moving to the mainland of the United States with a major increase in heart disease. It has also been shown that when the higher-meat diets of industrialized countries were adopted in less developed countries, the incidence of heart disease increased.

What about fats in plant foods?

There are many current myths about fats. That fats can play both a beneficial role *and* a damaging one is at the root of the confusion. If you have heart disease, you need to be extra careful about your animal fat intake. Making plant foods the centerpiece of your meals eliminates much of the worry about the amount of fat you take in—you'll automatically get the right kind of fat.

Remember that the fats in plants, with a few exceptions like coconut, are *good* fats. It is the fat from land animals—beef and chicken—that you need to be concerned about, because they contain large amounts of saturated fats. Natural plant fats are usually unsaturated. Furthermore, animal foods contain cholesterol, whereas there is no cholesterol in plant foods.

Aren't nuts high-fat foods that I should avoid?

Nuts are high in fat, but these are the good fats. Recent studies have shown that nuts help lower blood cholesterol, and in a major study done by Loma Linda University it was found that people who ate a few handfuls of nuts every week had fewer deaths from heart disease than people who did not eat nuts regularly. If you are on a plant-based diet, nuts supply good protein in addition to fiber and good carbohydrate. They also help you feel satisfied and prevent overeating because of the presence of their good fats.

Nuts, together with dried fruits like raisins, make great, healthful energy snacks. Trail mixes and many energy bars based on nuts, raisins, and other dried fruits are a great idea for anyone with heart disease. *Be sure the energy bar you choose contains no hydrogenated fats.*

Do you mean I can eat nuts and peanuts and use some olive oil?

It is difficult to overeat whole foods like nuts and seeds (for instance, sesame seeds, sunflower seeds, and peanuts) because the good fats they contain usually satisfy your hunger. Avocado contains good fats, as do soy and garbanzo beans. Cold-pressed oils like olive oil are full of good fats and antioxidants, and you can use them in moderation. (It is easy to overuse oils, and prolonged frying with any oil should be avoided, as the oil molecules in the fried food can be damaged by high heat.)

So, instead of thinking in terms of saturated or unsaturated fat, I should just think in terms of plant fat versus animal fat?

Yes. One of the few exceptions is coconut fat, which is not a good choice because it is very saturated. Just remember that there are two kinds of unsaturated fats: the monos and the polys, and that both are good for your blood cholesterol. The only common foods from plants that are somewhat saturated but have a fat that is neutral on blood cholesterol are chocolate and cocoa drinks. Olive oil and olives, which are mostly monounsaturated, have a long history of association with low heart disease rates in Mediterranean countries. Soybean oils found in tofu and many Asian foods have a similarly long history of association with low rates of heart disease in Japan, China, and Southeast Asia.

The choice is simple: eat your fat from plant foods, and limit your fat from animal foods by choosing either very low-fat or nonfat milk and other animal foods, or by using a higher-fat food like cheese only as a flavoring in very small amounts.

Is it true that not all unsaturated fats are good for me?

Yes. We have been talking about *natural* unsaturated fats. But problems creep up with processed unsaturated fats. When you take good polyunsaturated oils, like soybean oil, and make them solid, using a process called *hydrogenation*, the result is a mixture of fats that contain a certain amount of a "twisted" molecule. The natural state of this molecule is one of our safest fats, oleic acid, a monounsaturated fat. But the twisted molecules of monounsaturated fats are called *trans-fats* or partially hydrogenated fats or oils. (They are also called *trans-fatty acids*.) These fats are very common in foods because they are what the food industry calls *functional*: they work well in baked goods and many other products because they add texture and keep well. But through hydrogenation, the molecule has been changed enough to result in different physiological effects than our friendly soybean oil and nut fats. The world was shocked in 1990 when two researchers from the Netherlands, Drs. Katan and Mensink, published an article showing that these fats actually raise blood cholesterol and lower HDL, the good cholesterol.

How common are these trans-fats in supermarket foods?

These hydrogenated fats are so favored by the prepared food industry that they have made their way into French fries (one of the richest sources of trans-fats), other fried foods, breads and other baked goods, savory snacks, and many convenience and processed foods—like potato chips, corn and other chips, cookies, and crackers. For years they have slipped into our foods, and it was once thought that they were as good as the unsaturated fats from which they were originally made. A large study recently suggested that limiting consumption of trans-fatty acids would be more helpful in preventing heart attacks than simply limiting overall fat intake or even saturated fat intake.

It is a challenge to find ready-to-eat products without these fats added to them. Begin by avoiding foods that list "partially hydrogenated" oil or fat on the label. Margarine manufacturers are aware of this problem, so the old margarines that were based on partially hydrogenated oil are now slowly being replaced by margarines low in, or free of, these fats. Your best choice is to use some olive oil, avocado, and seed or nut butters like sesame, almond, or peanut on your bread instead of replacing butter with margarine—unless a careful reading of the margarine label shows little or no hydrogenated oil content or you use one of the cholesterol-lowering margarines.

How do I choose the healthiest kinds of meat, poultry, and fish?

Chicken, beef, pork, lamb, and other meats contain cholesterol and saturated fat. If you do eat them, choose the leanest parts and cuts. Remember that, per ounce, chicken with or without skin contains about as much cholesterol as red meat but is somewhat lower in saturated fat.

Between meat, poultry, and fish, fish should be your first choice. Even fatty fishes like salmon, tuna, sardines, and swordfish contain beneficial polyunsaturated oils. These oils help to lower blood triglycerides. These fishes are high in omega-3 fats. If your weight is a problem, choose low-fat fishes like sole, snapper, and halibut. Shellfish like shrimp and crab contain cholesterol but are very low in fat. Still, none of these foods should be the centerpiece of your meal.

Is it true that some fish fats are good for my heart?

Yes, they are not saturated like the fat from most land animals, and they also contain omega-3 polyunsaturated fats, which have unique protective properties, most notably preventing the formation of abnormal blood clots. It was as a result of research on Eskimos, who rarely developed problems related to abnormal blood clotting, that omega-3 fats became the focus of extensive research in recent years. Try to include some omega-3 fats from fish in your diet—especially from tuna and salmon. Unfortunately, about half of the salmon we eat comes from "farmed salmon," which contains much less of these omega-3 fats.

How can I get omega-3 fats if I don't eat fish?

Many plant foods also contain omega-3 fats. Good plant sources are flaxseeds, walnuts, grape seeds, pumpkin seeds, sesame, as well as some other plant seeds and their oils, and soybeans. They even occur in some leaves like purslane, a Mediterranean grass that grows wild in many parts of the United States. Include purslane in your diet, if you can find it or want to grow it!

What about very-low-fat diets?

Some studies have recommended a very-low-fat diet (20 percent or less of total calories) as a way to prevent atherosclerosis. These diets are typically high in carbohydrates (like grains, fruits, and vegetables), may include a small amount of animal-based foods, and severely limit fats of any kind. To succeed, these diets must include other important components of health such as intense physical activity, smoking cessation, and stress management. If you choose this kind of diet,

Table 11-2. Percentage of Saturated and Unsaturated Fat in Some Foods

Foods	Saturated fat	Unsaturated fat
Almonds	7	93
Beef	48	52
Butter and milk fat	66	34
Chicken fat	31	69
Coconut	92	8
Corn oil	16	84
Eggs (whole)	33	67
Flaxseed	10	90
Lard	43	57
Olives and olive oil	10	90
Peanut	19	81
Salmon	21	79
Sardines	22	78
Sesame seed and tahini	15	85
Walnuts	10	90

discuss it carefully with a health professional. To help prevent a rise in blood triglycerides, consume only whole grains. Keep refined grains, like white flour pastas and breads, to a minimum in this kind of diet. Some omega-3 fats should be included in such a diet.

What is the difference between refined and unrefined grains?

Grains, cereals, beans, nuts, and other seeds should be the cornerstone or centerpiece of a diet to support the health of your heart. However, for maximum goodness nutritionally and in taste and texture, they must be *unrefined*. You should limit your eating of white bread or cookies to rare occasions.

Historically, before the advent of roller milling in the late 1800s, which made it easy to produce the very white flour that is so prevalent today, populations ate hearty whole grains. These had flavor, texture, and all the natural, wholesome goodness that nature put into the grain. Even the white flour made from old stone mills and sifted at home to remove some of the bran was preferable to the white flour of today, as some of the bran and germ came through the old-fashioned sieves. The good fibers, proteins, vitamins like vitamin E, and minerals are in the germ or bran of the wheat. The wheat germ also contains a large number of newly discovered, precious phytochemicals that we are now finding are beneficial to health and that are absent from white flour. A wide variety of whole grain breads, pastas, and cereals is available today and there is no reason not to make them a key part of your diet.

For similar reasons, white rice is not the best choice. It has been polished and the fiber and B vitamins of the outer layer removed. It is the polishing of brown rice that caused an epidemic of the disease called beriberi in Asia. This was such a public health problem that, in the early 1900s, it led to the discovery of the first vitamin, thiamine or B_1, in the outer layers of brown rice. Barley, another ancient grain and a basic food in Roman times, is now polished to various degrees, again causing it to lose its fiber and vitamins.

No matter what grain you choose, always go for the whole grain!

Is it true that fiber lowers cholesterol and keeps me healthy?

It's true. There are many types of fibers found in plants, some of which lower cholesterol. The fibers found in oats, dry beans and lentils, dried peas, and fresh and dried fruits—like raisins—all lower cholesterol. Other fibers, such as those found in whole grains and their products like whole wheat bread and cereals, help to prevent constipation, improve intestinal function, and keep the colon healthy by reducing the likelihood of some diseases like colon cancer. Vegetables contain a mixture of both kinds of fiber.

There are some good fiber supplements, too. Many natural concentrated fibers like certain gums from plants, often with exotic names like guar, have been used in cholesterol-lowering supplements. Most of these supplements come in powder form and are based either on a single fiber like guar gum, pectin, or psyllium seed, or on a mixture of various gums. The easiest and probably the best way to take them is as a drink by stirring a tablespoon of the powder in a glass of cold water. The liquid tends to thicken after mixing, so drink it right away.

Can beans, soy, and lentils help me lower my cholesterol?

Yes, beans, soy, lentils, and peas contain the kind of fiber that can lower cholesterol. If you are not used to eating beans or lentils, you may experience some gas until you get adjusted, but there are so many varieties of beans and lentils that you are sure to find one that will not cause gas after you have eaten it for a few days. You may find it easier to start with lentils and its close relative the chickpea (also called garbanzo beans) and then begin to eat beans. Avoid beans prepared with saturated fat products like sausages as they often cause more gas.

Can food help me lower my blood homocysteine?

Folic acid, B_{12}, and B_6 are three B vitamins that help lower this risk factor, and the table below will guide you in selecting foods rich in each of them. Folic acid is on top of the list, and good sources are

Table 11-3. Food Sources of Folic Acid, Vitamin B$_{12}$, and Vitamin B$_6$

Folic-acid-rich foods	Vitamin B$_6$-rich foods	Vitamin B$_{12}$-rich foods
• leafy green vegetables like spinach, turnip and collard greens, green lettuce, and other green vegetables like asparagus and broccoli • lentils and garbanzo beans, navy beans, pinto beans, black-eyed peas, and other beans and peas • fortified cereals	• whole grains • bananas, green and leafy vegetables, potatoes, and watermelon • meat, fish, poultry • fortified cereals	• meats, fish, poultry, cultured milks like yogurt, other milk products, egg yolks • some yeasts • fortified cereals **Note:** vitamin B$_{12}$ is not found in plant foods

lentils, beans, dark green vegetables, and fortified breakfast cereals. It may be useful to take a supplement that contains these vitamins, as some people find it difficult to get enough folic acid from foods. Use either a complete vitamin-mineral supplement or a B-complex supplement.

What about those phytochemicals everyone is talking about?

Beginning in the 1970s with the discovery of the value of fiber and continuing in the late 1980s and 1990s with the identification of a long list of protective phytochemicals, our knowledge has grown far beyond the classic nutrition world of proteins, fats, carbohydrates, vitamins, and minerals. We have discovered that there are literally hundreds—and most likely thousands—of different compounds found in plant foods called phytochemicals (*phyto* comes from the Greek word for plant) that are biologically active in humans and animals. Just a few years ago, these compounds were thought merely to give color or flavor or to act as natural preservatives. Today we know that many of them help to prevent oxidation of blood cholesterol, which makes cholesterol more damaging.

Phytochemicals, like most everything else in nature and science, have complicated names, such as phenolics, flavonoids, phytoestrogens, and lycopene. However, they aren't usually listed on food labels. But the good news is that they all come packaged naturally, in nature's proper combinations, and in abundance when you make the right food choices. They work together with some powerful antioxidants, such as beta-carotene, vitamin C, vitamin E, zinc, and selenium.

Much research is still needed on the health benefits of the thousands of phytochemicals in unrefined plant foods, but you cannot go wrong by consuming an abundance of foods rich in phytochemicals.

What are the functions of antioxidants?

Antioxidants protect various compounds in the body from damage by some very active forms of oxygen, produced by various chemical reactions necessary to maintain body functions. Antioxidants protect cells exposed to toxic environmental factors, such as cigarette smoke, that cause cell damage, damage that can, in turn, contribute to the onset or progression of many diseases, including heart disease and cancer.

Should I take vitamin E to protect my heart?

In nature's design, this vitamin is actually a group of substances called tocopherols. They are found in abundance in plant foods high

---

FOODS RICH IN PHYTOCHEMICALS AND ANTIOXIDANTS

√• all fresh and dried fruits
√• all vegetables
• beans and lentils

• soybean products
• whole grains and their products
√• teas, especially green tea

in the good fats—almonds, wheat germ, whole grains, nuts, seeds, peanut butter, and in cold-pressed or minimally processed vegetable oils. Vitamin E and other tocopherols are powerful antioxidants, as well as vitamins. Like other antioxidants, they protect unsaturated fats from being damaged by oxygen. In humans, they help to protect against cell damage and damage to LDL. Some studies have also shown that vitamin E supplementation is associated with an increase in HDL and a reduction in LDL, and prevents abnormal blood clotting. Studies of various populations show that the higher the consumption of vitamin E, the lower the rate of heart disease.

First of all, get tocopherols from foods like whole wheat and nuts and seeds. Then you may consider a supplement, preferably of E with mixed tocopherols. A good choice is a 200-to-400-IU supplement. Closely related to vitamin E and the tocopherols are the tocotrienols, discovered a few years ago in barley and other whole grains. They lower blood cholesterol and are another piece of the body's antioxidant machinery.

How about vitamin C and heart disease?

Just as vitamin E is present in oils and other fats in plant foods, vitamin C is soluble in water and found in the many fluids of the body where water is the main component. It makes sense that vitamin C and vitamin E complement each other by working in different compartments of the body. For vitamin C, eat plenty of fresh fruits and vegetables—particularly kiwifruits, peppers, tomatoes, oranges, lemons and other citrus fruits, and dark green leafy greens. Supplemental vitamin C may help as well, as it is safe in moderation. But always make your vitamin C supplement a part of a diet high in antioxidants.

What about those yellow pigments found in carrots?

A wide array of colorful plant foods contain members of the carotenoid family. Beta-carotene is the most familiar to us, but there are actually many different carotenoids in nature. Some foods that are high in carotenoids are

- leafy greens such as kale, seaweed, spinach, turnip, collard greens, and mustard greens
- red, orange, and yellow fruits and vegetables such as apricots, cantaloupe, carrots, mangoes, papayas, peaches, red peppers, sweet potatoes, and winter squash

If you take a supplement of carotenoids, be sure it is not just isolated beta-carotene. All carotenoids have to work together. Only a few supplements contain them in combination, so read the label carefully before buying, and look for words such as "mixed carotenes."

Should I use herbs and spices in my cooking?

Yes. In all regions of the earth, kitchen herbs from rosemary to ginger and garlic have been used to flavor foods. Until recently, all we knew was that they helped us to enjoy our food and make it more flavorful. We came to associate sage and rosemary with Mediterranean cuisine, ginger with Indian cooking, and chili pepper with Mexican and Middle Eastern cooking.

But now we also know that all these herbs are extremely high in powerful antioxidants that prevent oxygen in the air from causing food spoilage or rancidity. Ginger added to foods in the hot climate of India helped to preserve food, as did sage and rosemary in southern Europe. Without knowing it, for centuries people were protecting themselves from heart disease and cancer by using these herbs and spices to preserve their food.

Garlic and its relatives in the onion family—onions, leeks, and shallots—contain powerful compounds that have antibiotic properties, that help control blood coagulation, and that, when combined with the proper diet, help to control blood cholesterol.

Use herbs, spices, garlic, and onions freely and regularly to add a pleasant form of protection to your meals.

Can I drink some teas, coffee, or cola beverages?

Yes, you may consume some caffeine-containing beverages; for example, two or three cups of tea daily. However, as caffeine is a stimulant that can increase heart rate, if you have arrhythmia, are prone to rapid heartbeat, or have high blood pressure, you should replace your caffeine beverages with decaffeinated beverages, preferably decaffeinated green tea.

The most common beverages or foods that contain caffeine are coffee, Indian and Chinese teas, maté in South America, and cola nuts, which gave their name to cola beverages. Don't forget that chocolate and cocoa products contain caffeine as well.

Green teas, and to a lesser extent black teas, are very high in antioxidants. Asian countries that have low rates of heart disease are typically tea-drinking countries. If you choose a beverage with caffeine, teas should be your first choice. Teas do not raise blood cholesterol.

Many cola beverages are based on caffeine and natural or artificial sweeteners, and do not contain protective phytochemicals. Recently some caffeine-containing soft drinks made from teas and other herbs have come onto the market; select these when you have a choice.

Coffee is not a rich source of antioxidants when roasted. Coffee does not affect blood cholesterol when brewed using a paper or metal filter. When it is made by boiling ground coffee, as is common in some countries, rather than by pouring boiling water over coffee grounds in a filter, it has been shown in some studies to raise cholesterol.

What about wine and alcohol?

Wine is a rich source of antioxidants, like other grape products. It also contains alcohol. Alcohol does raise HDL (good) cholesterol, and some studies have linked moderate wine consumption in countries like France and Italy to a lower incidence of heart disease. It is well known that alcohol should always be consumed in moderation and avoided during pregnancy. Perhaps the key to wine drinking is to consume wine only with meals. Even better, you may try diluting your wine with water, as is often done at Italian meals. The basic health rule is not to exceed one glass a day for women and two for men. Less research can be found on beer, but, again, a moderate amount may be beneficial. As with wine, if you choose to drink beer, do so with a meal. Drinking to excess may increase blood pressure and cause other health problems.

Recent reports about red wine show that it contains substances beyond the alcohol which have some extra benefits. A nondrinker can get those same benefits associated with red wine by eating grapes or raisins. It is the skin of the grapes (and raisins) that contains some of the antioxidants that seem to be responsible for the red wine effect.

This may be the reason why the French, even though their diet is high in animal fat, seem to have some protection against heart disease, protection not found in populations that eat similar amounts of animal fat but do not consume wine regularly. This is known as "the French paradox." The effect of wine, as with that of any other food, should always be considered in the context of the entire eating pattern. Mediterranean countries, like France, include large amounts of fruits and vegetables in their diet.

If you drink alcohol, your best choice is a wine with an alcohol content of about 11 to 13 percent, rather than higher-alcohol wines like sherry or port. Another good choice is beer, with an alcohol content of about 4 percent.

Is it true that the food I eat can interact with some of my medications?

Yes, some foods interact with drugs, and they may require the adjustment of dosages or other precautions. A tragic reminder is the death a few years ago of some patients on antidepressant medications called MAO inhibitors. When they ate aged cheeses or drank aged wines in an English hospital, some of them died. What caused their deaths was a compound called tyramine—innocuous to most—which raises blood pressure and is usually changed to a totally harmless substance in the intestines. But these medications blocked the activity of the compounds that performed this function and permitted tyramine to enter the systems of these sick people at full strength. Fortunately MAO inhibitors are used rarely since new antidepressant medications have become available.

Another example is grapefruit and grapefruit juice, which can interact with some drugs used to treat cardiovascular disease. Some compounds present in grapefruit interfere with the way the liver deactivates certain drugs. Be sure to tell your doctor or health professional if you regularly eat grapefruit or drink grapefruit juice. Otherwise, because of the inability of the liver to dispose of the drug in the normal way, the drug level could remain too high in the body.

Some vitamins may interact with other medications. For example, supplements or foods containing vitamin K may necessitate a change in anticoagulant medications. Foods may affect your drug needs and levels, *so be sure to tell your physician you are changing to this heart-healthy diet.* The dosages of some of your medications may need to be adjusted. (See Chapter 5, page 54, for a list of foods containing vitamin K.)

Is it true that a meal can kill?

If your coronary arteries are clogged, and if you have a tendency to form an abnormal blood clot (a *thrombus,* as described in Chapter 2), a high-animal-fat meal combined with low-fiber foods and refined carbohydrates can have consequences beyond the long-range effects we have seen. It can actually cause the formation of a clot in your coronary arteries, already clogged by plaques, and block them, causing a heart attack. If you have had a diagnosis of heart disease, you must be extra careful to avoid this type of meal.

We knew a heart disease patient in his late sixties, a former tennis pro, who had badly clogged coronary arteries. He used to be a regular smoker and ate a typical American diet. He had been warned to be extra cautious so as to prevent the possibility of major trouble, yet he neglected to follow simple guidelines about food and smoking. One Sunday morning he failed to show up for a tennis match he had arranged at ten. He had not forgotten the match. He had stopped at a coffee shop on his way and eaten a fat-laden breakfast. The meal caused a chain reaction that resulted in a blood clot forming in his coronary arteries that killed him.

Are there diets you can recommend?

The American Heart Association (AHA) diets are based on the principles we have talked about, with the primary focus being to reduce saturated fat and cholesterol. The National Cholesterol Education Program (NCEP) makes similar suggestions for dietary changes, so you may hear of an NCEP diet. AHA Step I Diet reduces saturated

THE ULTIMATE DESIGN
FOR A HEALTHY MEAL

(Some good recipe books are included in Suggested Reading, pages 140–52.)

The key foods for your main meals are from plants . . .

- GRAINS, whole wheat or whole grain breads, whole wheat pastas or pastas made with at least 50 percent whole grain and 50 percent semolina, brown rice, or other grains like barley and oats. Occasionally choose an exotic small grain like amaranth, teff, quinoa, or millet.
- BEANS, LENTILS, PEAS, to complement the grains. These legumes lower blood cholesterol and balance the proteins of grains. Don't forget soybean products like tofu, tempeh, miso, and soy milk.
- TREE NUTS, such as almonds, hazelnuts, pecans, walnuts, cashews, pine nuts, macadamias, pistachios, and their butters.
- SEEDS, such as sesame and sesame butter (also called tahini), peanuts and nonhydrogenated peanut butter, sunflower, and many other seeds and nuts. Nut milks.
- VEGETABLES of all types: some green leaves, like kale and collard greens, and dark green or red lettuces; roots like carrots, parsnips, and beets; tomatoes; peppers; squashes; broccoli and its relatives. Don't overlook artichokes, celery, fennel, and cucumbers.
- FRUITS of any kind, except coconut. Fresh whole fruits like grapes, figs, plums, cherries, berries—from raspberries to blueberries—citrus, kiwis, apples, pears, melons, and bananas. Dried fruits like sun-dried raisins and apricots. (Whole fruits are preferred over pieces.)

Of animal foods, your key choices are

- nonfat or low-fat cultured milks like yogurt or cheeses
- fish such as salmon, tuna, sardines, halibut, sole, or snapper
- lean chicken, baked, broiled, or boiled (chicken contains saturated fat and cholesterol, so use sparingly)

For flavoring, choose

- herbs, like sage, rosemary, ginger, chili peppers
- oils, like extra virgin olive oil and sesame oil
- vinegar, garlic, and small amounts of salt

---

fat to 8 to 10 percent of total calories and a Step II Diet reduces saturated fat to less than 7 percent of total calories. If you are accustomed to a typical American diet, to adopt a Step I Diet, you would need to reduce saturated fat by about one third, and for a Step II Diet you would need to reduce it by about one half. But don't forget: if you adopt a plant-based diet and cut down high- and medium-fat animal products, you'll be eating healthy without any complex calculations!

Can you give me a visual guide to choose my food?

We have created a new pyramid that we call the Healthy Heart Food Pyramid. In other food guide pyramids, the largest tier with the foods to be consumed freely as the foundation of the meal is at the bottom of the pyramid on tier one, and the foods to be consumed in very limited amounts are on the top tier. We have decided to put the foods that should be the basis of the diet on top, to draw your eye to the most desirable foods. The foods you should eat the least of are on the bottom.

Can I eat ethnic cuisines?

No matter whether you prepare meals at home or you eat out, ethnic cooking is a great way to have an appealing meal that never makes

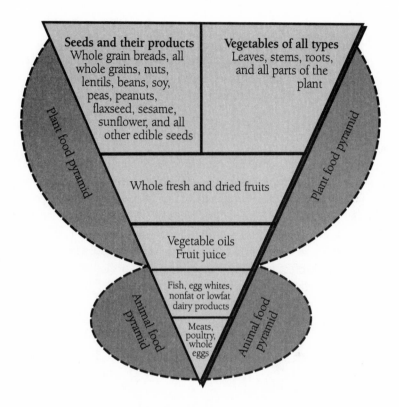

Figure 11.1. Healthy Heart Food Pyramid. Courtesy of the Sphera Foundation.

you feel you are on a "diet," and that offers tremendous variety. Choose Asian foods—avoiding monosodium glutamate (MSG)—like low-animal-fat Chinese, Japanese, and Indian; and low-animal-fat Greek, Italian, and Mexican foods . . . the list is almost endless. Remember that soy sauce can be high in sodium.

Always choose steamed and baked foods over fried; order tomato-based sauces over those prepared with butter and cream, or in Italian restaurants ask for olive oil; choose fish, tofu, and soup dishes at

Asian restaurants; and be sure to ask in Mexican restaurants for beans prepared without animal fat.

Should I take more time for my meals?

Remember Chapter 9 on stress? For centuries people, rich or poor, used to take the time to eat in a quiet environment. Dinner was an opportunity for a family to get together, to relax, perhaps to say a prayer.

In the modern world full of rush and stress, the time set aside for a peaceful dinner, prepared with love, has shrunk and often disappeared. A quickly defrosted, microwave-heated, precooked dinner eaten in a hurry is not uncommon. What should be reserved for an occasional meal in a special situation has often become a daily routine, just as a fast-food lunch has become the rule, rather than the exception, for many. There is a place for all of this, but a quiet meal, with no pressure—what we call *the meal ritual*—should be part of a healing and protective day for anyone, but even more so for someone with heart disease. This not only is important to allow you to prepare superprotective foods but is a key component of stress relief.

If you can devote some time to relaxation before your meals—even a few minutes—this will make your meal ritual even better.

Epilogue

Today, with our knowledge of heart disease, we can unequivocally say that your future health, and perhaps your life, is in your hands. Some simple concepts can make a tremendous difference not only in your health but in your quality of life—whether you have been diagnosed with heart disease and want to prevent a possible heart attack; have had a heart attack, are now on your way to recovery, and want to prevent a second heart attack; have a major risk factor like high blood cholesterol; or, just as important, you do not yet have heart disease but have a family history of heart disease.

Which of the keys to heart health is the most important?

Your entire lifestyle is important: avoid thinking only in terms of diet or exercise or stress relief or smoking cessation. They all work together in a way that will surprise you. Making positive changes in any of these areas will be helpful, but never forget that the way to fuller health is to eliminate all the risk factors and add all the protective factors.

Learn to think in terms of total lifestyle rather than isolated actions! Too many people concentrate on just one heart disease risk or protective factor, maybe avoiding smoking or cutting down on saturated fat, or exercising more or doing some relaxation exercises. These are all good things to do, but in isolation they are not sufficient. Think of a total lifestyle change.

However, a gradual stepwise approach is usually best, working on one risk factor at a time. The sense of victory and self-confidence you will gain from eliminating one risk factor will lead to better success in conquering the other risk factors.

How can I visualize the ultimate heart disease prevention lifestyle?

Visualize all the protective factors as part of a team rather than as isolated entities, with all of them working together to make you healthy and keep you that way. Read over and over again Chapter 3 on the risk and protective factors. Make a copy of the Lifestyle Pyramid and the Healthy Heart Food Pyramid (page 137) and keep them where you can refer to them daily.

Can this lifestyle help prevent other chronic diseases?

Yes! A lifestyle that can prevent heart disease is the same lifestyle that can keep your body in better condition, decrease your chance of developing osteoporosis (bones becoming brittle in aging), prevent hip fractures, decrease the chance of cancer, and allow you to retain youthful vitality and avoid other problems as you get older. This healthy lifestyle is important for people with heart disease, but it applies to everyone. Food choices, exercise, weight control, and avoiding stress and cigarette smoking all form the foundations of healthy living.

How can I succeed at my new lifestyle?

To succeed, make your new lifestyle a joyful, pleasant experience. This is a point too often overlooked in learning new lifestyles. If each step is a chore, you won't stay with it very long. If your heart disease has not yet gone too far, think how drug-free and surgery-free you could be: both drugs and surgery may become a necessity if you do not do something now. If you have survived a heart attack, unless you enjoy your new lifestyle, you'll slowly switch back to your old

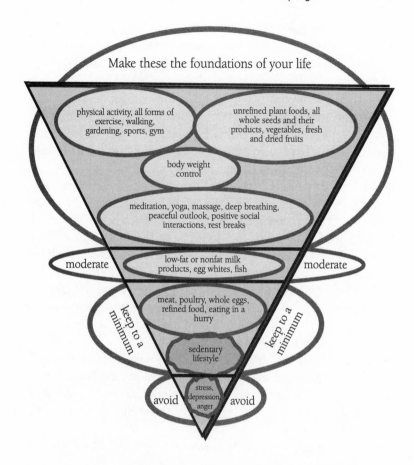

Figure 12-1. Lifestyle Pyramid. Courtesy of the Sphera Foundation

habits. If you have to be on medications, consider how much more enjoyable it would be to be able to decrease their dose, their number, and the risk of adverse effects, and perhaps someday not need these medications at all.

How do I make my new lifestyle a joy instead of a chore?

There are some dos and don'ts. Let's briefly revisit them; then you may want to go back and reread the chapters on the specific topic.

- Never say or think "I am on a diet." The term diet makes you think of restrictions, hospitals, somebody watching over you and telling you what to do. *You are not on a diet, you are enjoying foods at their best and you prepare them the way you like them. Nothing has more flavor than real, whole foods.* It's too bad the term diet has taken on such a negative meaning. That's why, in this book, we have avoided the term as much as possible. No diet for you! Soon you'll say: "I have to go out to dinner. I hope they have the food I love"—your new foods, that is!

- Never say or think "I must exercise now." Rather, think what a lift you'll get from physical activity. Make it a habit, so that soon you'll say, "I am taking a walk during my lunch break at work, it makes me feel so good." It should be a chore *not* to do it! Seize any chance for physical activity. Never take a motorized vehicle when you do not need to. If you play golf, never take that golf cart. If a store is within walking distance, walk to it. If you can take the stairs instead of an elevator, do so. If you can use a manual lawn-mower, don't use a motor-driven one. Make it a habit. Enjoy being outside and reducing the stress of driving.

- Never say or think "I have no time for my meditation or a break." Everyone can find a few minutes at home or at the office, even on a busy day. It will give you renewed energy and make the rest of the day easier. Soon you'll say, "I feel so great after doing it, I want to do it more often."

- Never let anger, depression, or fear take over. Use that energy to exercise or, if you feel the need, see a therapist.

- Never say or think "I have to live by this and that rule." There are no rigid rules for you, rather a joyful search for the ultimate healthy way of life. Rules are made to be broken, but joy is here to stay.

A final word . . .

Put an aura of joy around your new lifestyle, the joy of your new state of well-being, far beyond what you have ever experienced. In an era when people look to drugs to solve every minor problem, you are now on a path where drugs play their proper role: they should be used with care to treat major diseases or problems and not as a substitute for a healthy lifestyle. When you look back a few years from now, with your heart disease a memory of the past, you'll say, "It's so simple, I never enjoyed life so much. Why doesn't everybody follow this path?"

Glossary

adjuvant therapy: See **combination therapy**.

adverse effects or side effects: Harmful, undesirable effects of a medication or treatment procedure.

aerobic exercise: Exercise where oxygen is used, such as jogging, hiking, bicycling, or swimming.

angina (angina pectoris): Chest pains due to coronary heart disease: "stable angina" if it comes at predictable times over a few weeks; or "unstable angina" if the pain comes at rest, is more severe, or increases in duration (over ten minutes) or frequency. Unstable angina is a signal that you need to seek immediate medical attention, as it may be the warning symptom of an impending heart attack.

angio-: A prefix that means blood or lymph vessels.

angioplasty: Use of a thin tube with a balloon tip to unblock a coronary artery, also called percutaneous transluminal coronary angioplasty (PTCA).

aorta: A large artery that arises from the left ventricle and brings fresh blood to the body.

arrhythmia: A disordered rhythm of the heartbeat which can be fatal (see **ventricular fibrillation**) but which usually is not life-threatening, especially if it originates from the upper chamber of the heart, or *atrium*.

artery: Any one of the small and large blood vessels that carry oxygen and nutrients to all parts of the body.

atherectomy: Physical removal of plaque from coronary arteries.

atrial fibrillation: A type of arrhythmia centered at the upper chamber of the heart.

blood cholesterol: A fatlike substance produced by the liver, an important building block of cells and a precursor of various hormones.

blood triglycerides: Common fats in the blood, used by the body for energy.

blood vessel: Any one of the vessels that carries blood, such as arteries and veins.

bypass: See **coronary bypass surgery**.

CAD: See **coronary artery disease**.

cardiac: Related to the heart.

cardiomyopathy: Another cause of congestive heart failure (CHF) which occurs most often in adults, preceded by many months of shortness of breath; a problem not due to atherosclerosis and most often with no known underlying cause.

cerebral thrombosis: A blood clot that forms, completely blocking an artery in the brain.

CHD (coronary heart disease): Same as coronary artery disease (CAD), but a more frequently used term.

combination therapy: A therapy combined with another for increased effect.

congestive heart failure (CHF): The inability of the heart, as a pump, to maintain the circulation of blood.

cooling-off period: Slowing down after intense physical activity rather than suddenly stopping.

coronary arteries: The arteries that feed and bring oxygen to the heart muscle, and the clogging of which leads to heart disease.

coronary artery disease (CAD): See **coronary heart disease**.

coronary bypass surgery: Surgical grafting procedure that bypasses a clogged coronary artery by attaching a clean blood vessel from another part of the body.

coronary heart disease (CHD): Degenerative and metabolic changes of the coronary arteries, usually due to formation of plaque.

diastolic blood pressure: The lower value when measured when the heart is dilated and resting for an instant between beats (from the Greek *diastellein*, "to dilate").

embolism: A small fragment of atheroscelerotic plaque that plugs an even smaller artery in the brain.

fibrates: Drugs that primarily lower triglycerides.

heart attack: See **myocardial infarction.**

high-density lipoprotein cholesterol (HDL): Known as the "good," or heart-protective, cholesterol.

homocysteine: An amino acid that, if elevated, can damage muscles and make blood susceptible to forming clots.

hypertension: High blood pressure.

infarct or infarction: A sudden insufficiency of blood to a region of the heart.

lipoprotein: A term derived from *lipo,* which means fat, and protein.

low-density lipoprotein cholesterol (LDL): Known as the "bad" cholesterol, linked to coronary heart disease risk.

myocardial: Referring to the myocardium; see **myocardium.**

myocardial infarction: Damage to a small or large area of the heart muscle.

myocardium: Heart muscle.

niacin: A B vitamin that, in large amounts, lowers cholesterol.

percutaneous transluminal coronary angioplasty (PTCA): See **angioplasty.**

plaques: Deposits of cholesterol and fibers in the inner wall of arteries.

resins: Drugs that bind bile acids.

resistance exercises: Exercises that bear weight against muscles, like weight lifting, which work well together with aerobic exercises.

rheumatic heart disease: A disease caused by late effects of an earlier infection with the streptococcus bacterium; more common fifty years ago, before antibiotics were available; causes damage to one or more of the heart's valves.

statins: Drugs that inhibit cholesterol production.

stent: Implant to make an artery opening wider and prevent it from narrowing again.

stretching exercises: Exercises designed to stretch the muscles of the legs, arms, and abdomen before strenuous exercise; important to help prevent injuries.

stroke: Injury to a part of the brain caused either by bleeding from a brain artery or from a blockage of a brain artery. Strokes caused by bleeding from a tear in the brain's arteries are called hemorrhagic strokes and are particularly common in those with high blood pressure.

synthesis: Preparation of a compound from simpler compounds or elements, either in nature or in a manufacturing process.

systolic blood pressure: The higher value when measured at the peak of the heart's contraction (from the Greek *systellein,* "to shorten").

total blood cholesterol: The total cholesterol (HDL, LDL, and VLDL) found in the blood.

transient ischemic attacks (TIAs): Often also simply called "small strokes" to indicate that their effects are often brief, usually lasting less than an hour.

valves (heart valves): Membranous structures that open and close to let blood in and out of the four chambers of the heart.

vascular: Relating to blood vessels.

vena cava, superior: The large vein that brings blood back to the heart after it has circulated through the head and neck, upper limbs, and thorax. Sometimes just called vena cava.

ventricular fibrillation: A rapid quivering of the lower heart chambers (the ventricles) which can only last for a few minutes before death occurs.

very low-density lipoprotein (VLDL): One of the lipoproteins that carries cholesterol in the blood.

warm-up period: A period of easing into a strenuous exercise session to reduce the chance of injury.

APPENDIX B

Suggested Reading

Health

American Heart Association Guide to Heart Attack Treatment, Recovery, and Prevention. American Heart Association. New York: Times Books, 1996.

The American Way of Life Need Not Be Hazardous to Your Health. John W. Farquhar. Menlo Park, N.J.: Addison-Wesley, 1987.

Anger Kills: Seventeen Strategies for Controlling the Hostility That Can Harm Your Health. Redford Williams and Virginia Williams. Scranton, Pa.: HarperCollins, 1998.

Cardiac Rehabilitation: Clinical Practice Guideline Number 17. U.S. Department of Health and Human Services. AHCPR Publication no. 96-0672, 1995.

Cardiac Rehabilitation: A Guide for Patients. Robert F. DeBusk. San Ramon, Calif.: Health Information Network, 1996, series no. 0113.

Cardiac Rehabilitation as Secondary Prevention: Quick Reference Guide for Clinicians Number 17. U.S. Department of Health and Human Services. AHCPR Publication no. 96-0673, 1995.

Coronary Bypass: A Guide for Patients. Timothy A. Denton and Jack M. Matloff. San Ramon, Calif.: Health Information Network, 1997, series no. 0112.

50 Essential Things to Do When the Doctor Says It's Heart Disease. Fredric J. Pashkow and Charlotte Libov. New York: Plume/Penguin, 1995.

The Feeling Good Handbook. David D. Burns. New York: Plume/Penguin, 1990.

Heart Disease: How to Work with Your Doctor and Take Charge of Your Health. Mike Samuels and Nancy Samuels. New York: Summit Books, 1991.

Heart & Soul: A Psychological and Spiritual Guide to Preventing and Healing Heart Disease. Bruno Cortis. New York: Pocket Books, 1995.

How to Reduce Your Risk of Heart Disease. John W. Farquhar and Prudence E. Breitrose. San Ramon, Calif.: Health Information Network, 1994, series no. 0111.

The Last Puff. John W. Farquhar and Gene A. Spiller. New York: W. W. Norton, 1990.

Natural Medicine for Heart Disease: The Best Alternative Methods for Prevention and Treatment. Glen S. Rothfeld and Suzanne LeVert. Emmaus, Pa.: Rodale Press, 1996.

The New Living Heart. Michael E. DeBakey and Antonio M. Gotto, Jr. Holbrook, Mass.: Adams Media Corporation, 1997.

Palpitations and Arrhythmias: A Guide for Patients. Nora Goldschlager. San Ramon, Calif.: Health Information Network, 1997, series no. 0115.

Recovering at Home with a Heart Condition: A Practical Guide for You & Your Family. Florence Weiner, Mathew H. M. Lee, and Harriet Bell. Howard A. Rusk Institute of Rehabilitation Medicine. New York: Body Press/Perigee, 1994.

Triglyceride, High Density Lipoprotein, and Coronary Heart Disease. National Institutes of Health Consensus Statement, 1992.

Yoga: 28 Day Exercise Plan. Richard Hittleman. New York: Workman Publishing, 1975.

Nutrition

Note: The cookbooks in this list all contain excellent recipes, but you may need to modify some of them to reduce the amount of salt they contain, as well as saturated fat and cholesterol from milk, cheese, and egg yolks.

The Art of Chinese Vegetarian Cooking. Joanne Hush. Rocklin, Calif.: Prima Publishing, 1996.

Asian Vegetarian Feast. Ken Hom. New York: Quill/William Morrow, 1988.

The Barm Baker's Book. Monica Spiller. Los Altos, Calif.: Sphaera Press, 1992.

The Book of Miso. William Shurtleff and Akiko Aoyagi. Berkeley, Calif.: Ten Speed Press, 1989.

The Book of Tempeh. William Shurtleff and Akiko Aoyagi. New York: Harper & Row, 1985.

The Book of Tofu. William Shurtleff and Akiko Aoyagi. Berkeley, Calif.: Ten Speed Press, 1998.

The Chile Pepper Book. Carolyn Dille and Susan Belsinger. Loveland, Colo.: Interweave Press, 1994.

Chinese Vegetable & Vegetarian Cooking. Kenneth H. Lo. New York: Faber & Faber, 1995.

The Complete Book of Herbs and Spices. Sarah Garland. New York: Viking, 1979.

Couscous and Other Good Food from Morocco. Paula Wolfert. New York: Harper & Row, 1973.

Diet for a Small Planet. Frances M. Lappé. New York: Ballantine, 1986.

Eat Your Way to Better Health: Good Health and Great Recipes with the Super-pyramid Eating Program. Gene Spiller. Rocklin, Calif.: Prima Publishing, 1996.

The Grains Cookbook. Bert Greene. New York: Workman Publishing, 1988.

Great Meatless Meals. Frances M. Lappé and Ellen B. Ewald. New York: Ballantine, 1984.

The Greens Cookbook. Deborah Madison and Edward Espe Brown. New York: Bantam Books, 1987.

Healthy Nuts: Your Guide to the Healthful Benefits of Nuts. Gene Spiller. New York: Avery Putnam, 2000.

Herbal Renaissance. Steven Foster. Salt Lake City, Utah: Gibbs Smith, 1984.

Lean Bean Cuisine. Jay Solomon. Rocklin, Calif.: Prima Publishing, 1995.

Lord Krishna's Cuisine: The Art of Indian Vegetarian Cooking. Yamuna Devi. New York: Bala Books/E. P. Dutton, 1987.

Lorna Sass' Complete Vegetarian Kitchen. Lorna Sass. New York: Hearst Books, 1992.

The New Soy Cookbook. Lorna Sass. San Francisco: Chronicle Books, 1998.

Not Milk . . . Nut Milks! Candia Lea Cole. Santa Barbara, Calif.: Woodbridge Press, 1990.

Nutrition Secrets of the Ancients: Foods and Recipes for Optimum Health in the New Millennium. Gene Spiller and Rowena Hubbard. Rocklin, Calif.: Prima Publishing, 1996.

Recipes from an Ecological Kitchen: Healthy Meals for You and the Planet. Lorna J. Sass. New York: William Morrow, 1992.

Recipes for a Small Planet. Ellen B. Ewald. New York: Ballantine, 1986.

The Rice Book. Sri Owen. New York: St. Martin's Press, 1993.

The Savory Way. Deborah Madison. New York: Bantam Books, 1990.

The Superpyramid Eating Program. Introducing the Revolutionary Five New Food Groups. Gene Spiller. New York: Times Books, 1993.

Vegetarian Cooking for Everyone. Deborah Madison. New York: Broadway Books, 1997.

Vegetable Heaven. Mollie Katzen. New York: Hyperion, 1998.

Verdura: Vegetables Italian Style. Viana La Place. New York: William Morrow, 1991.

▬

Sample Medication List

Week of _____

Time	MEDICINE	Dose	Sun	Mon	Tue	Wed	Thu	Fri	Sat

Index